1991

W9-ADS-742

3 0301 00055959 7

Medical Ethics:

Common Ground for Understanding
Volume II

Kevin O'Rourke, OP, JCD
Dennis Brodeur, PhD

LIBRARY
College of St. Francis
JOLIET, ILLINOIS

The Catholic Health Association
of the United States

Copyright © 1989
by
The Catholic Health Association of the United States
4455 Woodson Road
St. Louis, MO 63134-0889

Printed in the United States of America. All rights reserved. No part of the publication may be reproduced, stored in a retrieval system, or transmitted, in any form or by any means, electronic, mechanical, photocopying, recording, or otherwise, without the prior written permission of the publisher.

Library of Congress Cataloging-in-Publication Data

(Revised for volume 2)

Medical ethics.

   Includes bibliographies and indexes.
   1. Medical ethics.   2. Physicians — Professional ethics.   3. Medical ethics — Case studies.   I. O'Rourke, Kevin D.   II. Brodeur, Dennis.
R724.M2942   1986   174'.2   85-21349
ISBN 0-87125-109-4 (v. 1. : pbk.)
ISBN 0-87125-145-0 (v. 2. : pbk.)

G
174.2
O75
2

Table of Contents

140, 433

Introduction

During the past few years, medical ethics has become "everybody's business." The ethical implications of such issues as genetic engineering, surrogate motherhood, in vitro fertilization, and the AIDS epidemic go beyond the research laboratory, the hospital, and the long term care center. The ethical decisions made in regard to these contemporary research and medical procedures will determine for years to come what kind of people we shall be and what type of society we shall create.

The time is far past when scientists and healthcare professionals were the only persons responsible for ethical decisions regarding research and medical care. To paraphrase the famous proverb concerning the responsibility for decisions about war, medical ethics is too important to be left in the hands of scientists and healthcare professionals. Thus, although we stress the responsibilities of scientists and healthcare professionals in these essays and articles, we realize that these issues dramatically affect all persons in society. We address these reflections to a wide spectrum of society, realizing that persons with many different talents must be involved in the decision-making process that will direct medical research and healthcare.

The first volume of *Medical Ethics: Common Ground for Understanding* resulted from our efforts to build an education and research program in healthcare ethics at the St. Louis University Medical Center (SLUMC). This second volume contains some of our efforts directed to the same goal, but it also reflects our attempts to serve a wider audience, namely, healthcare professionals and interested persons from every occupation across the United States. Thus, some articles in this volume are essays written for the SLUMC community; others were written for people serving on institutional ethics committees (IEC) and appeared in *Issues: A Critical Examination of Contemporary Ethical Issues in Health Care,* a publication of the SSM Health Care System. Still other selections were published in scientific and healthcare journals or in publications intended for a general audience.

In short, these writings represent our efforts to reach a wide audience and to present and apply ethical principles to contemporary problems and issues arising from scientific research, medical practice, and healthcare delivery.

The essays and articles in this volume are directed toward people living in a pluralistic society. Although not in conflict with the Catholic traditions concerning medical ethics that both authors represent, the selections offered are based on a logical and reasoned approach to the issues considered. We do not question or reject a faith commitment to the Catholic Church's teaching regarding research and medical issues, but we seek to substantiate our considerations in a way that speaks to all people in our pluralistic society.

Our ethical considerations are based mainly on two objective realities that are validated by mutual human experience: (1) the needs that human persons have in common, and (2) the goals of medicine as evidenced in the physician-patient relationship. One will find in these writings frequent references to the physiological, psychological, social, and spiritual needs of the human person. Achieving the fulfillment of these needs in a balanced manner is the purpose of ethics. Moreover, it will become clear that although medicine and healthcare in the strict sense are concerned with only the first two needs of the human person, the physiological and psychological, medicine and healthcare in the *ethical* sense must consider the other two human needs as well: the social and spiritual. The purpose of healthcare and medicine is understood ethically only if the full spectrum of human needs are considered as integral elements of the human person seeking healthcare.

The equality of persons in the physician-patient relationship will also be an underlying theme of this volume. The equality of persons is not predicated on equal medical knowledge, but rather on the dignity and worth of each human person. Thus, although these articles are directed toward a pluralistic society, we draw on a very definite concept of the human person and some precise values and goals of the healing relationship. We believe that this concept of the human person and the values inherent in the patient-physician relationship are the basis for ethical analysis, as validated by common experience. Furthermore, we believe that this concept and these values have been well suited for the healing professionals and have brought out the best in healthcare professionals over the centuries.

The essays are gathered in three general sections with no reference to the time at which they were written. Part one contains those essays examining the concept of medical ethics for a pluralistic society and expressing some thoughts on the physician as ethicist. While we center upon physicians as the audience and subject of some essays, we include implicitly other healthcare professions. Thus, what is predicated on or directed to physicians applies *mutatis mutandis* to nurses, hospital administrators, people in allied healthcare professions, trustees, and those in any way associated with healthcare.

Part two considers some general principles of medical ethics. The consideration of principles is not taxonomic; rather, we present some of the more important principles, seeking to ground medical ethics in values and objective reality as opposed to opinion and erroneous concepts of the human person.

Part three considers cases that have been prominent in the media, as well as critiques of articles that have appeared in medical journals. While we do not always seek to solve the cases in question because information sufficient for an informed ethical decision is seldom presented in the media, we do seek to present the principles that should be utilized in answering similar questions that might arise in the course of offering healthcare. In response to the journal articles, we seek to consider the assumptions upon which they are based, to analyze the reasoning of the articles, and to state the implications of the conclusions when these are ethically significant for healthcare professionals.

Finally, our thanks are due to the people at St. Louis University Medical Center and the SSM Health Care System who have supported us in our programs of education and research, especially to Arthur E. Baue, MD, vice president of SLUMC, and to Sr. Mary Jean Ryan, FSM, president and chief executive officer of SSM Health Care System. Special gratitude is due to our friends and assistants, Judy Diggs, Donna Callis, and June Granville, who have helped prepare these manuscripts for publication.

Medical Ethics and Professional Responsibility

Part I

Medicine: 1
Not an Exact Science

Across the United States, compensation is sought for injuries suffered in the course of medical care. In an effort to control medical insurance rates, to limit the size of awards from injuries, and to improve the quality of medical practice, New York and other states are revising the laws regarding damages resulting from medical care and regarding certification of physicians. Although some action is needed to limit the extent of the "malpractice mess," many of the solutions apparently are based on a false notion of medicine and healthcare. To provide some light in this heated discussion, a more accurate notion of medicine and medical judgments seems necessary.

Principles

Medicine is not an exact science. An exact science is a body of knowledge that allows one to reach certain conclusions from causes and to apply that knowledge without fear of error. Mathematics is an exact science. Only human error causes defects in mathematical conclusions. Although medicine applies exact sciences—for example, it relies on the sciences of anatomy, biochemistry, or pharmacology—medicine applies knowledge gained from exact sciences to particular people. Medicine aims primarily at the well-being of individual persons. Thus, the specifying element of all knowledge and techniques of medicine is the *individual* for whom the knowledge and techniques are used. Medicine is relativized because of this orientation.

Moreover, consider that medicine is concerned with preventing illness and with curing illness. In both cases, medicine cannot formulate specific norms that are certain to apply for all people or express ineluctable diagnoses or prognoses. When prevention of illness or disease is in question, the potential for framing scientific norms or regulations is impossible. Some even maintain that the "science" of preventive medicine has been so overrated as to destroy its worth.[1] One can improve one's well-being to some extent through regimen and discipline and perhaps limit the possibility of contracting certain diseases, but no definite connection exists between lifestyle and avoiding disease. Although one may never have smoked cigarettes, this is no guarantee that one will never contract lung cancer.

In regard to curing illness, the intrinsic causes of uncertainty and error are even more prevalent and serious. First, individuals are different in their physiological makeup. Thus, medical diagnosis and prognosis are not precise and exact. Through their bodies, human beings may be studied and objectified. From this objectifying, general scientific conclusions about health, disease, and etiological agents of disease may be drawn. The uniqueness of each human person, however, which is expressed in the individual's body, cannot be generalized and objectified. The response of each patient to therapy cannot be predicted scientifically. The "art of medicine" is operative when science is applied to the individual. Because the physician assumes responsibility to help the patient strive for health, medicine is a unique form of art because its "work" is a better human being, not merely an improved inanimate object. The uniqueness of each human body is illustrated in all therapies, but most especially in the use of pharmaceutical compounds. Even though drugs are tested through clinical trials for adverse effects before their approval by the Federal Drug Administration, the search for harmful side effects after approval must continue because pharmacological compounds affect different people in different ways.[2] Penicillin, for example, serves as a forceful antimicrobial agent for most people, but for some people it triggers a toxic or allergic reaction that may be fatal.

A second factor limiting the certainty of medical judgments is the difficulty in obtaining sufficient empirical evidence to guarantee the certainty of the medical diagnosis. The anatomy of a clinical judgment combines inductive and deductive reasoning and is filled with uncertainties. Symptoms may be similar for several illnesses or diseases. Moreover, even if laboratory tests are used in making a diagnosis, they may vary widely in reliability and accuracy. Thus, even if tests are available and symptoms abound, the diagnosis of an illness is tentative. One conclusion may be more probable than another but far from certain because the "right" information might be unobtainable. In sum, the process of reaching a diagnosis is dialectical, not the result of rigorous scientific reasoning. The potential for misdiagnosis is evidenced by autopsy studies that show the correlation between the cause of death and the clinical diagnosis is far from exact.

Finally, another cause for uncertainty and ambiguity in medical decision making is the value system of the patient. Medicine is primarily concerned with the patient's physiological well-being, but this in turn is directed to the individual's social and spiritual (cognitive-affective) good. In other words, although physiological health is a foundational value of human life, it is not the only value. A patient may have some social or spiritual values that will determine the type of medical treatment he or she chooses to receive. Thus, the "right" physiological therapy for a particular person may not always coincide with the patient's value system. The person suffering from cancer may determine to forego curative or palliative treatment in order to devote his life savings to his children's education rather than to therapy that may or may not be successful. The importance of the patient's value system and its influence on therapeutic choices is a vital element in medical decision making. Clearly, it is another source of uncertainty in reaching therapeutic conclusions.

Discussion

Why do people believe that physicians are able to make completely accurate diagnoses about illnesses and infallible decisions about healing therapies for various diseases? Why does the general public, especially members of juries, usually presume that "someone has to pay" if a patient suffers an injury in the course of medical care? Pellegrino and Thomasma[3] attribute this prevalent mistaken notion about medicine to Cartesian dualism. Descartes separated the person and the body, seeking mathematical certainty in medicine. As a result, however, he introduced a false dichotomy that presented the human body as a machine, an entity that could be disassembled and repaired like other machines. This concept dehumanizes medicine. Also, one must admit that the medical profession has not sought avidly to dispel the aura of infallibility surrounding it.

Given the intrinsic uncertainty of medical decision making, therefore, plans to evaluate physicians because of their "mistakes" are unsound. Attendance at continuing education programs may be required of physicians, but it is unjust to measure medical acumen by counting "mistakes" or malpractice accusations. Mistakes resulting from patient neglect or physician impairment should be declared as such and just compensation offered. For this reason, physician review boards should be composed of consumers as well as professionals. A contract of justice exists between physician and patient, and the physician is held to make restitution if he or she does not fulfill the object of the contract. But the contract's object is not a certain scientific diagnosis or prognosis. Rather, this contract is a dialectical decision founded on scientific knowledge but influenced by the particular physiology of the body; the ambiguity of symptoms, signs, and tests; and the differing value systems of individual persons.

Conclusion

Applying the foregoing concepts will not eliminate all problems arising from medical practice. The perspective of the general public, legislators, judges, and juries, however, may be more accurate if they realize (1) medicine is not an exact science, and (2) physicians make judgments that "follow the rules" but that still may be inefficacious. In their diagnosis and prognosis, physicians may be in error through no moral, cognitive, or technological fault of their own.

1. Lenin Goodman and Madeleine Goodman, *Hastings Center*

Report 16:2, April 1986, pp. 26–27.
2. Gerald Faich, "Adverse Drug-Reaction Monitoring," *New England Journal of Medicine* 314:24, June 12, 1986, pp. 1589–1592.
3. Edmund Pellegrino and David Thomasma, *A Philosophical Basis of Medical Practice,* Oxford University Press, New York, 1981, p. 99.

Medical Decision Making   2

Peter Marzuk wrote "The Right Kind of Paternalism"[1] in a 1985 issue of the *New England Journal of Medicine,* one week after Norman Cousins' "How Patients Appraise Physicians"[2] was published in the same journal. There are notable similarities in their articles that draw attention to the psychodynamic and interpersonal elements of communication in the patient-physician relationship. As medicine develops and technology progresses, people become more knowledgeable (or fearful) of technology. This less quantifiable, less empirical dimension of medicine requires greater attention.

Marzuk points out that underlying emotional dimensions of illness may cloud the ability of a patient to make appropriate decisions. Hidden agendas of anger, fear, denial, or depression may result in noncompliance with or outright defiance of the physician. Some time and energy by the physician must be devoted to unmasking these blocks to good decision making by the patient. Respect for autonomy should not push the physician to collude in decisions against the patient's self-interest. "To accede easily to ill-advised patient decisions in the name of patient autonomy is not to enhance medical consumerism. It is just bad medicine."[3]

In the other article Cousins reports on a very unscientific survey of an upper middle-class neighborhood. One thousand survey forms were distributed to a residential area requesting written answers to three questions (plus self-addressing the return envelope and paying for the postage!). 586 forms were completed and returned. Of these, 85 percent reported they had changed their personal physician during the past five years or were presently contemplating making a change. Twenty-five percent of these did so because they perceived their physician to be incompetent, but the bulk of respondents changed physicians because of personality and communication issues.[4] Although the verbatim responses are interesting, the underlying theme is that patients have expectations about communication, dissemination of information, and other "difficult to measure" interpersonal skills.

Both articles are cause to reflect on the values of patient

autonomy, the skill of communication, informed consent, and public health education.

Principles of Good Decision Making

In recent years, informed consent has received much attention in medicine, law, and ethics. Legal concerns often predominate, but the underlying ethical issue is to provide a patient with an opportunity to participate in medical decision making to the fullest extent possible, respecting autonomy and self-determination. This is accomplished through the patient's voluntariness, ability to reason, comprehension of the nature of the illness, and ability to weigh the various risks and benefits of each alternative therapy available, including doing nothing. When all factors are present, the patient's choice should be respected. The values of autonomy and self-determination have received greatest attention by philosophers and some medical professionals. However, exclusive emphasis on these two dimensions blurs the basic goals of medicine and good medical decision making.

Each element of informed consent has underlying assumptions that must be examined. Voluntariness or patient freedom may be the most difficult. Assuming a patient is competent, unless otherwise contraindicated, is different from the assumption that illness so incapacitates a person that he or she could not make any decisions. Categories of patients considered to be incompetent should be reexamined. Minors and people suffering from depression or dementia are often capable of making some healthcare decisions. Voluntariness is not a black and white issue and therefore demands time from the physician.

The ability to reason has several assumptions as well. One is closely akin to the competency issue. First, some people can grasp medical issues, which implies appreciation, knowledge, and deep understanding of medical realities at an early age or when suffering from serious illness. Others, even when adult and healthy, cannot. Second, processing information for decision making requires biological knowledge. Knowing something about organ systems, the way the human body functions and reacts, is vital. Often this knowledge does not exist, making the education task more difficult. In addition, the ability to appreciate how medicine is practiced is crucial. Generic words such as "cancer" often hide the facts of a particular malignancy and the possibilities of successful treatment. Misconceptions about the "science" of medicine confuse patients when other people with the same disease have different outcomes.

When informed consent requires the ability to reason and to balance risks and benefits of various alternatives, a complicated process is taking place. Simple solutions that place all alternatives before the patient with the expectation that a choice be made (under the guise of autonomy) or that presumes patient ignorance (thus promoting paternalism) are unacceptable. It is in this area that the two journal articles clearly command attention. Uninformed autonomous decisions mask foolishness on the part of the patient, and unprofessional conduct on the part of the physician. Paternalistic decision making by the physician violates the patient-physician relationship.

Patients usually come to physicians because they are no longer capable of taking care of themselves. They lack the knowledge and skill necessary to take appropriate action. Communication is therefore vital. One form of communication is educational. Physicians unable to educate well may not be able to help patients make beneficial decisions. However, other educators, nurses, healthcare professionals, family, and friends may be helpful in this endeavor. Counseling skills are another form of communication. Psychotherapy is not a required skill, but a fundamental sense of the basic principles of general counseling is required. Emotional, familial, and social problems may prevent beneficial decision making. Helping a patient cast aside these stumbling blocks is necessary to promote good health and autonomy. Paternalism connotes a tainted image today, but this cannot overshadow the need for physician guidance in decision making.

Conclusion

Cousins' informal survey points to patient expectations about physicians' ability to communicate. He ends his article by pointing to the surplus of physicians, implying that these issues demand attention in a period of abundance in the supply-demand elements of contemporary economics. If, however, the ethical and medical realities of informed consent are taken seriously, it is not the overabundance of physicians that should command attention, but rather the quality of the patient-physician relationship and the demand of excellent medical decision making, regardless of the number of physicians.

1. Peter M. Marzuk, "The Right Kind of Paternalism," *New England Journal of Medicine* 313:23, Dec. 23, 1985, p. 1474.
2. Norman Cousins, "How Patients Appraise Physicians," *New England Journal of Medicine* 313:22, Nov. 28, 1985, p. 1422.
3. Marzuk, p. 1576.
4. Cousins, p. 1423.

Various Ethical Systems 3

Why do different people arrive at different solutions to ethical problems in medicine, even if they begin with the same set of facts? Why, for example, do some persons, whether physicians or family members, decide it is an act of mercy to remove artificial nutrition and hydration from a patient in an irreversible coma, whereas others would maintain that the same action would be murder? One reason for disparate ethical decisions is because people use different ethical systems in reaching decisions about right and wrong actions. In this essay, we describe briefly the various systems that people use to reach ethical decisions. Then we evaluate these systems according to their effectiveness in a pluralistic society.

Ethics seeks to determine which actions will contribute to a person's fulfillment or happiness. Ethics presupposes human freedom and human responsibility. When judging which actions to perform, such as whether to gain money by stealing or through work, a person often faces a conflict. One action is good from one point of view: stealing is an easier and often quicker way of obtaining money. The other action, however, is good from another point of view: working enables one to retain personal integrity, respect the rights of others, and avoid the disgrace associated with theft. How do people settle the conflict? Whether they realize it or not, people use a consistent method of ethical decision making when they are faced with such questions. The major systems of ethical decision making are:

1. *Emotivism.* This ethical theory relies mainly on subjective, emotional response. According to this theory, something is right or wrong because "I feel it is right or wrong." In the United States today, this method of ethical reasoning is widespread. Many will defend their own or others' ethical choices as long as the people making decisions are "sincere." This method of decision making leads to exaggerated individualism, as Robert Bellah and others demonstrate in *Habits of the Heart.*[1] Although emotions are an important factor in making good ethical decisions, by themselves emotions alone do not offer a sufficient basis for developing a system of shared values in a pluralistic society. Moreover, emotivism does not enable one to measure an

action in accord with one's human fulfillment, unless one maintains emotional satisfaction is the same as human fulfillment.

2. *Legalism.* This ethical system maintains that the law determines what is ethical. In healthcare, this method is often used with a view toward avoiding malpractice litigation. Thus, physicians, hospital administrators, trustees, and their legal advisors often ask, "What will help us avoid malpractice?" rather than, "How do we foster patient benefit (fulfillment)?" This method perverts the relationship between ethics and law. Laws should be founded on ethical norms, but the law often falls behind ethical thinking. For example, to assert that artificial hydration or feeding cannot be removed unless there is a law enabling people to do so ignores the essential goal of fulfillment of persons through medical care. Thus, laws are helpful if they express sound ethical norms, but laws are not the ultimate norm for ethical choices in a pluralistic society.

3. *Cultural Relativism.* This ethical method decrees that actions are ethical if they correspond to the customs of a society or a segment of society. Simply because people are accustomed to performing actions, however, does not mean this is an ultimate judge of these actions' ethical worth. Probably the most significant examples of cultural relativism for the healthcare professions are found in the various codes of ethics used by different associations. For example, the American Medical Association's Code of Ethics approves of some actions that are in themselves unethical and disapproves of others that are not unethical. However, no substantial reasons are given for the decisions offered. Does one have to follow the codes in question to be a good physician? In the past, the codes of ethics for physicians have contained blatant violations of patients' rights, especially in regard to informed consent.[2] Thus, customs and codes are only worthwhile if they are subject to more basic ethical evaluation. Something is not ethical in our pluralistic society simply because "everyone does it."

4. *Fideism.* This method of ethical decision making is based upon religious faith in a church or a person. Although church directives may be helpful and fulfilling for human beings, and although many churches offer worthwhile and reasonable explanations for their teachings, the ultimate motivation for

accepting the teaching is religious faith. Thus, directives of churches, even though reasonable, will not be accepted in a pluralistic society by people who do not share the same faith.

5. *Reasoned Analysis.* This method judges ethical issues by reasoning about the effect of the action on the important values of life and the consequences of the action on persons involved. This system seeks to discern whether or not the action and its consequences contribute to human fulfillment and happiness. Reasoned analysis in ethical investigation is difficult and intricate because it means one must seek some common definitions pertinent to human fulfillment and happiness. It also means one must formulate general norms concerning human functions and human values in order to guide decision making.

Reasoned analysis in ethical decision making is complicated and intricate, but it has been successful in the healthcare field because many norms have been accepted in regard to ethical healthcare. For example, all accept that medical personnel should obtain informed consent before treating patients because this disposes for human fulfillment. Moreover, it is accepted that life-support systems may be removed if they are useless or involve a grave burden to human fulfillment. Likewise, most accept that access to healthcare for poor people is a public concern. The many volumes published by the President's Commission for Protection of Human Subjects and the President's Commission for the Study of Ethical Problems in Medicine and Biomedical and Behavioral Research are examples of the effort to approach ethics through reasoned analysis.

Although agreement exists on many major ethical issues in medicine, we do not mean to imply that all ethical issues are near solution. The ethical evaluation of abortion is one area in which consensus has not materialized. We do insist, however, that reaching consensus in our pluralistic society on abortion and other converted ethical issues is not possible unless a process of patient and comprehensive examination of the ethical issues occurs through reasoned analysis. Only through this method can consensus be developed concerning actions that foster or impede human development. And only then will we have the opportunity for consensus in our pluralistic society.

Conclusion

A number of books describe in detail the various ethical systems. This brief synopsis presents a general idea of each system and why we often differ on ethical conclusions, even though we may begin with the same set of facts.

The next time you seek to make an ethical judgment or are involved in an ethical debate, analyze the method of decision making that you are using. Realize that some methods are not well-founded because they do not ask the basic questions. Also, realize or recall that for our pluralistic society we need a method of ethical decision making founded on the reasoned analysis of shared values.

1. Robert Bellah et al., *Habits of the Heart,* Harper & Row Publishers, New York, 1985.
2. Carleton B. Chapman; *Physicians, Law, and Ethics,* New York University Press, New York, 1984.

Who Will Determine   4
Medical Ethics?

Court cases show the confused state of affairs in regard to the ethics of medicine. The Supreme Court of New Jersey, in the famous Claire Conroy case, determined that tube feeding could be withdrawn from a comatose patient if severe pain is present or there is some indication that the patient would choose removal of life-support systems were he or she able to do so. Later, in Dedham, MA, a probate judge issued an injunction blocking the removal of tube feeding from Paul Brophy, a comatose firefighter, who had expressed a desire to die swiftly in case of severe disabling illness. The judge, in face of the realization that no therapy would restore Brophy's cognitive functions and discounting Mrs. Brophy's and her children's request to terminate life support, declared that "it is ethically inappropriate to cause the preventable death of Brophy by the deliberate denial of food and water which can be provided to him in a noninvasive, nonintrusive manner which causes no pain and suffering, irrespective of the substituted judgment of the patient."[1] This trial court decision was later reversed by the Supreme Court of Massachusetts.

Principles

Clearly, the courts are in disagreement because no accepted ethical norm in medicine exists for the treatment of persons who are in a vegetative state. Should life-prolonging therapy be withdrawn if cognitive function cannot be restored? Is nourishment furnished by tube feeding necessary only for comfort, or is it only a life-prolonging therapy? Or is it both comforting and life-prolonging and/or comfort therapy? There is no well-reasoned, commonly accepted, moral imperative offered by physicians in this regard.

Although we wish to express our dismay at the decision of the court, we would attribute the cause of the confusion to the medical profession rather than to the legal profession. An intricate relationship exists between ethics and law: legislation and judges should express and protect existing ethical principles when they make decisions. Their proper mandate is not to formulate ethical norms, but rather to apply them. Law and court decisions should be founded on ethics, not vice versa. Both law and ethics imply an obligation to follow the norm stated by either discipline. The obligation of law usually involves a material penalty of one type or another; a fine or incarceration results if one violates a legal obligation. The obligation of ethics is one of conscience. Even though violating ethical norms may not involve material loss, one's integrity and authority are weakened or lost by violating ethical norms. Skeptics may state that ethics is less important than law because violation of law implies more definite penalties, but the professions, especially the profession of medicine, have always valued integrity and honesty above material goals.

Why are physicians in the United States reluctant to state ethical norms before the courts and legislatures do? What prevents physicians from agreeing on ethical norms that would serve as the basis for ethical obligations, laws, and legal decisions? Several viewpoints seem to prevent physicians from assuming this form of leadership:

1. As Carleton Chapman pointed out in a recent work of outstanding insight and scholarship, "some physicians view medicine solely as bioscience."[2] Physicians of this mentality are more concerned with protecting their own prerogatives than they are with the delineation of the moral purposes of medicine and the rights and obligations that arise from the patient-practitioner relationship. Chapman proposes that this mentality has dominated the ethical statements of the American Medical Association for more than 100 years.

2. Although some physician groups have sought to state principles of medical ethics, their efforts have not been forceful enough. Physicians are reluctant to admit that ethical norms

involve "should" and "ought"; that is, that they oblige in conscience. Thus, the American College of Physicians commissioned an ad hoc committee to formulate some principles of medical ethics.[3] The committee prepared a reasoned text considering many different cases and the ethical principles usable in different situations, but the principles were submitted as *guidelines*. Ethical principles are not guidelines, if this means, as it usually does, that one is morally free to accept or reject these principles. Ethical principles are more than guidelines. Until physicians admit that ethical principles are norms that imply a "should" or "ought" in medical practice, all ethical statements will lack credibility and effectiveness. The "ethics as guidelines" mentality was reflected in a recent statement of the American Hospital Association (AHA). After approving a set of objective norms for ethical patient care, the Board of Trustees of the AHA stated: "By definition, there are no objectively right or wrong answers to the dilemmas generated by conflicting values."

By opting for ethical norms that imply moral responsibility, we are not implying that detailed norms can be stated for every case and that a "cookbook" of ethical actions could be published. Rather, we maintain that a set of norms could be developed by physicians that, in the words of the President's Commission on Ethics in Medicine, would contain "substantial rules identifying the various factors that look to ethically defensible decisions and which suggest procedures that would make careful considerations of these factors more ikely."[4] Thus, some statements of ethics fail not because they are too particular, but because they are put forth as suggestions or guidelines instead of objective norms that involve moral obligations.

3. Finally, some statements on medical ethics fail because the physicians do not utilize the help of ethicians and philosophers. Recently, a group of physicians sought to state norms for ethical treatment of "hopelessly ill patients" and failed to distinguish the ethical difference between patients who are "hopelessly ill" and those who are merely "pleasantly senile."[5]

Statements of medical ethics will never have any force in medical and legal circles unless they are formulated by physicians. The basis for such formulations should be a reasoned analysis of the purpose of medicine and the responsibilities of the physician-patient relationship. In the formulation of ethical norms for medicine, however, physicians should be aided by those who have expertise in ethics and philosophy.

Conclusion

"The medical profession has never developed a forum within its structure that is suitable for the systematic discussion of such items (i.e., ethics) and as a consequence has been handicapped in many ways through the centuries."[6] In these words, Chapman indicates that physicians, in their professional societies, must pave the way for the formulation of ethical norms for medicine. In the words of another physician, "The point is that we physicians must be the ones to decide how we practice our profession."[7] If physicians do not decide the ethical norms for the profession, then legislation and the courts will continue to decide for them.

1. *Patricia E. Brophy vs. New England Sinai Hospital Inc.*, The Trial Court; Norfolk, MA; N85E0009-G1.
2. Carleton Chapman, *Physicians, Law and Ethics,* New York University Press, New York, 1984, p. 147.
3. American College of Physicians' Ad Hoc Committee, "American College of Physicians' Ethics Manual, Part I" 1984:101, 129–137, "American College of Physicians' Ethics Manual, Part II," 1984:101, 263–274, *Annals of Internal Medicine* 101, 1984, pp. 129–137.
4. President's Commission for the Study of Ethical Problems in Medicine and Biomedical and Behavioral Research, *Summing*

Up, U.S. Government Printing Office, Washington, DC, 1983, p. 66.

5. Sidney Wanzer et al., "The Physician's Responsibility Toward Hopelessly Ill Patients," *New England Journal of Medicine* 310:15, Apr. 12, 1984, pp. 955–959.

6. Chapman, p. 159.

7. Charles Davidson, "Are We Physicians Helpless?" *New England Journal of Medicine* 310:17, Apr. 26, 1984, p. 117.

The Limits of Patient Autonomy   5

Patient autonomy has reached benchmark status in most ethical reflections on healthcare. After years of discussion and expansion of patient decision making, however, many providers have begun to ask: Has the benchmark been set too high? Can there never be cases when "doctor knows best"?

Today's patients have a right to accept or reject any medical treatment. Physicians, nurses, and healthcare facilities continue to struggle with such ideas as a patient's right to refuse or to withdraw from any medical treatment, the professional's obligation to continue treatment, and the legal ramifications of withdrawing or withholding treatment.

Many reasons underlie the concern expressed about the principles of informed consent, proxy consent, the values of patient autonomy, and the mechanisms used to ensure patient rights. Most are related to the last few decades' development of informed consent as a legal issue and patient autonomy as a positive value.

Institutional ethics committees (IECs), increasingly have discussed these issues as they relate to questions of death and dying, adults and neonates, competent and incompetent patients, and physically and mentally ill persons. Most discussions, however, have centered around the idea that the patient or his or her proxy should hold ultimate, decision-making authority. Healthcare professionals now are discovering that this presumption may not always be in the patient's best interest.

The Question of Futility

Various articles in medical journals recently have addressed this issue with titles such as, "Survival after Cardio-Pulmonary Resuscitation in Babies of Very Low Birth Weight: Is CPR Futile Therapy?"[1] "Must We Always Use CPR?"[2] and "Interpreting Survival Rates for the Treatment of Decompensated Diabetes: Are We Saving Too Many Lives?"[3] Each article addresses basic problems of cardiopulmonary resuscitation (CPR) and do-not-resuscitate (DNR) orders. This gives rise to the question: Has the ascent of patient autonomy as an almost sacrosanct value in healthcare ethics glossed over deeper problems of useless treatment?

For example, one article documents the cases of low-birth-weight neonates, those less than 1,500 grams, who suffer from other associated medical problems and fail to survive CPR after experiencing cardiac arrest.[4] Should standard procedure require that neonates under certain birth weights not be resuscitated when other related health problems exist? Should a DNR order be obtained from the parents even though medical professionals know the treatment will be futile?

Similar questions about whether or not CPR should always be administered are raised in another article[5]: Are there clear medical indications that some CPR attempts are certain to be futile? If so, is CPR really an option? How can CPR be justified when it will not benefit the patient?

Consensus Lacking

Ethical problems arise because there is a lack of consensus about useless treatments not having to be offered or accepted, especially in the case of CPR, DNR orders, and other so-called life-sustaining procedures.

Certain precedents support the notion that useless treatments do not have to be offered to some individuals, regardless of their health status. The Chad Green case in Massachusetts, for example, confronted physicians with the question of whether they had to offer the boy's parents the option of using the drug laetrile to treat his leukemia, as the parents wished. Because laetrile has no proven efficacy in treating leukemia and is not accepted in the United States, the physicians' consensus was that laetrile treatment did not have to be offered. Later, after Chad's parents sought laetrile treatment for him in Mexico, they were faced with accusations of child abuse.[6] Why should CPR, when proven ineffective, be any different from so-called quack treatments such as prescribing laetrile for leukemia?

IECs can deal with these questions in a variety of ways. Committees that focus on education can benefit an institution simply by discussing the problem. Those that facilitate policy making can lead the move toward refining policies to allow physicians the decision-making latitude required by quality care. Committees that provide consultative services may be called on to help outline options and potential outcomes in specific cases. Some requests for consultation may be based on a family's insistence on treatments that will not benefit an incompetent patient. Both physicians and IEC members must be prepared to grapple with family requests that may be based on emotional or social difficulties experienced at a critical time in life.

What Constitutes Useless Treatment?

First, ethics committees must clearly define "useless treatment." An article previously cited divides useless treatments into three categories:[7]

1. Treatment that will neither save nor promote a person's life

2. Treatment that may save physiological life but produce an unacceptable quality of life where an acceptable quality of life existed previously

3. Treatment that will save a physiological life whose quality already is unacceptable

The first category can be illustrated by the cases of low-birth-weight neonates who suffer from other complications and die, as expected, even after CPR. Despite the most noble attempts to provide medical care to such infants, CPR likely will not save their lives. Even if it does, they will live only briefly before undergoing another cardiopulmonary event or succumbing to their other medical problems or complications of the CPR attempt. The question is whether or not CPR should be tried at all, and whether standing DNR orders should be initiated for infants who suffer from such problems.

This category is not exclusive to infants. For example, many adults who suffer from coronary disease associated with other major organ failures, high blood pressure, or additional problems will not benefit from continued CPR. Numerous studies have examined CPR's effectiveness in certain patient populations. How should healthcare institutions handle these issues?

The second category of useless treatment encompasses people who are satisfied with their present quality of life but who fear that CPR or any other major medical intervention will merely prolong their physiological life at a quality they cannot accept. Although these individuals may reject the notion of CPR, they may wish to have other aggressive treatment performed to preserve their present quality of life from problems not associated with cardiac arrest.

This raises the often-asked questions about what DNR orders really mean. Can a patient whose chart contains a DNR order still be aggressively treated in the intensive or cardiac care units? Can a person with a DNR order undergo surgery that may be beneficial as long as cardiac arrest does not occur? In these cases, useless treatment is defined in part by each patient's subjective preference for a quality of life presently obtainable but presumed unattainable in the event of cardiac arrest and "successful" CPR.

The third category of useless treatment is represented by those who believe their present quality of life is unacceptable and who would welcome death. They reject not only CPR, should cardiac arrest occur, but also any other lifesaving procedures. Whether death results from cardiac arrest, pneumonia, or another problem that could be ameliorated briefly is insignificant. DNR orders are simply an expression of the fact that continued aggressive medical treatment to save their present lives is not acceptable to them.

Subjective Interpretation

All three categories just discussed involve different interpretations of useless treatment. Each situation must be addressed uniquely and with great care, because these decisions made by patients cannot be equivocal or ambiguous.

IECs that seriously approach their charge to help develop policies surrounding death and dying or the refusal of medical treatment must be clear about what can be considered useless treatment. They must assess the consequences of administering identifiably ineffective medical treatments while considering patient's wishes to continue or reject treatment. In doing so, IECs must ask: Does adherence to the principle of patient autonomy require that people be accorded a right to choose useless treatments?

This can be a complicated issue, especially when discussed from the perspective of patient preferences for certain treatments, whether or not these are beneficial. The simple truth is that some treatments will not benefit some patients regardless of individual values. IECs need to address whether or not physicians and institutional policies can require that patients explicitly reject medically useless treatments. Committees also must consider whether physicians are free to enter into a discussion about why a certain treatment will not be ordered regardless of the patient's or guardian's expressed wishes.

This is clearly apparent in DNR orders. If all scientific evidence in the medical profession points to the fact that certain individuals will not benefit from CPR, must a physician treating this patient still require patient or proxy consent before entering a DNR order? Should the physician be ethically bound to explain to the patient or proxy that CPR will be useless and that a DNR policy will be followed regardless of the patient's wishes? Or should the physician initiate discussion with the patient about a useless treatment and be obliged to follow patient choices regardless of the possible benefit?

Difficulty in Communication

Any of these alternatives raises emotional and ethical issues for the patient. Each also raises questions about the communication mechanism used by the physicians, nurses, institutions, and other healthcare providers to help patients understand the CPR endeavor.

A fundamental issue germane to these discussions is that of patient-physician communication. The process, which is not an easy one to begin with, grows more complicated as patients

LIBRARY
College of St. Francis
JOLIET, ILLINOIS

become incompetent and proxy decision makers with their own emotional agenda enter into the discussion.

Degree of difficulty aside, these issues still must be raised, and the IEC can be an ideal forum in which to raise them. Discussion should cover useful and useless medical treatments, patient rights and patient autonomy, and the type of physician and other professional care necessary for good medical decision making. As inconclusive as these discussions may be, they serve as a warning against trying to cover too many technical subjects under the general theme of patient autonomy vs. efficacy of lifesaving treatments, such as DNR orders, pulmonary assistance, expensive antibiotics, or surgery.

Another temptation is to equate DNR orders and rejection of other lifesaving treatments with the idea of simply allowing a person to die. These are separate notions that may not always mean the same thing. A patient who asks not to be resuscitated may request other kinds of aggressive treatment. A physician who places a DNR order on a patient's chart may still continue ICU care and other aggressive treatments in the hope that the patient, who considers present quality of life acceptable, will not suffer cardiac arrest. Because each case can be so different, institutional policies must allow for nuance and interpretation.

Conclusion

Institutional policies concerning patient autonomy must provide guideposts and not recipes for medical treatment. This requires careful assessment of patient values, physician and other healthcare provider judgments, and social policy. Ethics committees can contribute to the discussion of the role of patient decision making and medical care in a way not available through any other sector of the healthcare environment. Maturing IECs can begin to address some of these deeper ethical issues by recognizing (1) that fine distinctions must be made to ensure patient rights and autonomy are respected, (2) that latitude for good medical judgment is created, and (3) that institutions reflect the values most significant in caring for patients with life-threatening illnesses.

1. John D. Lantos et al., "Survival after Cardiopulmonary Resuscitation in Babies of Very Low Birth Weight: Is CPR Futile Therapy?" *New England Journal of Medicine* 318:2, Jan. 14, 1988, pp. 91–95.
2. Leslie Blackhoel, "Must We Always Use CPR?" *New England Journal of Medicine* 317:20, Nov. 12, 1987, pp. 1281–1285.
3. John Yudkin, Ian Doyal, Brian Harwitz, "Interpreting Survival Rates for the Treatment of Decompensated Diabetes: Are We Saving Too Many Lives?" *The Lancet,* 1987, i, pp. 1192–1195.
4. Lantos et al., p. 92.
5. Tom Tomlinson and Howard Brody, "Ethics and Communication in Do-Not-Resuscitate Orders," *New England Journal of Medicine* 318:1, Jan. 7, 1988, pp. 43–46.
6. *In re Green,* 282 A. 2d 387 MA. 1972.
7. Tomlinson and Brody, p. 43.

Two Ethical Approaches   6
to Research on Human Beings

Since World War II Catholic Church and national and international study groups have issued separate sets of statements regarding the ethics of scientific studies involving human beings. The Church refers to this topic as "experimentation on human persons," whereas the study groups describe the topic as "research involving human subjects." Whichever term is used, it means seeking generalizable knowledge concerning human function or behavior through empirical studies.

After considering the areas of agreement and disagreement in the two sets of statements, a look at the ethical foundations for the statements may foster a better understanding of the important ethical issues arising from research involving human subjects.

Areas of Agreement

The Catholic Church's statements and the study groups' documents set forth many similar ethical norms for research involving human subjects:

1. Research on human subjects, because it yields knowledge that benefits individuals and society, is a vital part of scientific medicine and should be fostered and promoted.[1]

2. Ethical research requires the informed consent of the subject or a guardian or proxy. Informed consent requires the subject's knowledge, understanding, and freedom.[2] The Church and study groups both approve double-blind studies and the use of control groups, provided the subjects are notified beforehand that one segment will not receive the substance or procedure under study.[3] The study groups have insisted more strongly on review boards to protect subjects from unwarranted harm and risk and to ensure that the subject is truly informed.[4] The Church is more inclined to leave the researchers responsible for protecting subjects and obtaining informed consent.[5]

3. Research on human subjects is therapeutic or nonther-

apeutic.[6] Therapeutic research, either standard or innovative, aims at bettering the subject's medical condition. Standard therapeutic research deals with practices that have been accepted as safe and helpful, such as research involving the use of beta blockers to control hypertension. Innovative therapeutic research deals with practices that have not yet been accepted as standard, such as the initial research on the left ventricular assist device as a means of restoring cardiac function. A medical procedure or mechanical device used as part of a research program must be evaluated under two formalities: whether it contributes to the physiological or psychological well-being of the patient, and whether it yields generalizable knowledge. The significance of the distinction between therapeutic and nontherapeutic research is seen principally in assessing legitimate risk for oneself or another.

4. The risk of harm involved in research must be evaluated in regard to the potential benefit intended by the procedure in question.[7] If the research is therapeutic, one may agree to participate even though some risk of harm is foreseen. If the research is nontherapeutic, one may put oneself at risk for other people provided the risk is reasonable and freely accepted.[8]

The Church statements base the evaluation of risk and benefit on the principle of double effect. According to this principle, the action that could lead to risk and harm must be performed with the intention of healing the patient. Moreover, the action must be designed in such a way that it has the potential to accomplish that intention.[9] Thus, when performing open heart surgery, the surgical team intends to repair the arteries to supply blood to the heart. If harm occurs, it arises from a cause beyond the intention of the surgical team and beyond the design of the surgery. It occurs as an undesired and indirect result of the surgery.

The study groups imply a utilitarian judgment of risks and benefits, which inclines toward assessing results alone, rather than the agent's intention and the act's design.[10] Utilitarian reasoning states: "The action is ethical because more good than harm results from it." The knowledge of human morphology, for example, could be increased considerably by nontherapeutic research on human embryos. But in the course of this research, living embryos would be destroyed. Because living embryos are human beings, the Church maintains the actions that destroy them intentionally and directly are unethical.[11] The study groups look to the beneficial results of such nontherapeutic research and declare it to be ethical.

5. The case is somewhat different for proxy consent.[12] If the research is therapeutic, the proxy may subject the incompetent person to risk or harm as long as hope exists for proportionate benefit to the person. Parents may consent to serious surgery for an infant, for example, if the surgery may be deemed therapeutic. But because proxy consent is designed to protect the incompetent person's well-being and humanity, the proxy may expose a ward to only "minimal" danger or harm in nontherapeutic research.[13] Minimal harm or risk is that associated with routine medical testing.

6. Research on human beings should be allowed only after appropriate research on animals.[14] Although animals should be treated humanely and should not be exposed to unnecessary pain or death, research on animals is ethical.[15]

7. Researchers should practice equity in selecting subjects and scientific problems to be studied. Society must protect its weaker members, such as the retarded, prisoners, and the poor.[16] Moreover, researchers must not select scientific projects only to enrich themselves.[17]

8. The human subject or proxy should be free to withdraw from the research program at any time.[18]

Some of the assumptions underlying the Church and study group statements may lead to different practical applications of these principles. When both the Church and the study groups require informed consent to protect the "dignity of the person," for example, the Church bases its view of human dignity on the belief that man and woman are made in the image and likeness of God, whereas the study groups' documents usually base their view on the principle of autonomy.[19]

The principle of autonomy is not contradictory to Church teachings, but it does not emphasize the person's natural need of community as the Church teachings do. Moreover, the Church presupposes that the goal of human existence is eternal life, whereas the study groups usually do not. (Eternal life means there is life after death. This must be factored into an ethical analysis. If one's concept of autonomy, for example, does not envision eternal life, one will have a limited view of autonomy and make decisions accordingly.) Finally, although both groups require proxy consent, the purpose may differ. The Church statements assume that the proxy will help the incompetent patient toward eternal life, whereas the study groups wish to protect the person's autonomy.

Areas of Disagreement

The Catholic Church expresses unmitigated opposition to nontherapeutic research on embryos.[20] The Church also has serious reservations about genetic research that results in changes in the human body or mind. "It is really of great interest to know whether an intervention upon the genetic store exceeding the bounds of the therapeutic in the strict sense is morally acceptable," states Pope John Paul II. He then lists conditions of ethical genetic research, the most important being respect for the body-soul unity of the human person. He concludes: "Such an intervention must consequently respect the fundamental dignity of mankind and the common biological nature which lies at the basis of liberty; respect consisting in the avoidance of manipulations tending to modify the genetic store and to create groups of different people, at the risk of provoking risk marginalizations in society."[21]

Although study groups realize that genetic experimentation is dangerous because the results are unpredictable, they express a willingness to undertake such experiments because the anticipated knowledge will be useful.[22]

The study groups are divided regarding nontherapeutic research on human embryos. The Australian Study Group rejected such research,[23] but the study groups in the United States,[24] the United Kingdom,[25] and the report on the International

Bioethics Summit Conference[26] approved it in principle, even though the human subjects might die as a result.

The International Bioethics Summit Conference maintains: "There is a need *to keep in balance* [emphasis added] the professional liberty for clinical treatment and for scientific inquiry in the interest of progress in medical knowledge and skill while upholding regard for the human interest of the embryo."[27] The study groups stated that embryo research is acceptable if a review committee approves it. The review committees recommended in contemporary studies, such as the Warnock Report, are concerned primarily with balancing, not protecting, the subject's rights. The review committee, representing a cross section of the public as well as scientific interests, seems to have the responsibility of reflecting public opinion, not of judging the ethical merit of the acts in question.[28]

The Church and the study groups also disagree on the use of in vitro fertilization and embryo transplant to initiate pregnancy.[29] This disagreement primarily regards the use of "spare embryos" resulting from in vitro fertilization, the use of third-party donors of ova or sperm for in vitro fertilization, and the circumvention of intercourse in generation.[30]

Ethical Foundations

A complete analysis of the differences underlying the two statements would require a resume of the history of philosophy and an accounting of the differences between faith and reason, but some explanation of the differences is possible. The Church's traditional theology and philosophy maintain that some human actions are good or evil in themselves, as determined by objective evidence.[31] This objective evidence is derived from studying the human person's nature and purpose, which requires considering the needs, functions, and bodily integrity of the human person. (The relationship of functions of the human person are explained in the principle of totality—an important element in medical ethics proposed by the Church.[32]) Thus researchers should consider not only the extrinsic effects (results) of the human act when evaluating moral action, but also the intrinsic effects, which signify the act's impact on the person who performs it or on whom it is performed.

The intention and the result of the action are significant factors in the ethical evaluation. If the action is evil insofar as the natural needs and functions of a person are concerned (its intrinsic effects), it is not ethically good simply because it results in a good effect. Some of the Church's ethical norms—for example, "do not kill innocent human beings"—do not allow exceptions because the human acts they prohibit are evil for everyone.[33]

The study groups, on the other hand, seem to have changed their grounding for ethical statements. Immediately after World War II, the foundation for ethical research involving human subjects was, in one form or another, Kantian autonomy, with several exceptionless norms stated.[34] The postwar declarations were designed to correct the evils resulting from relativistic ethics.

Recent statements from the study groups, however, follow a utilitarian grounding.[35] According to this ethical approach, which is common in our society, no actions are good or evil in themselves, no exceptionless norms exist, and an action is good as long as the person performing the action believes "it results in more good than harm."[36] Thus, the question asked in many contemporary studies of ethics and human research is whether the research results in more good than harm. If it does, the research is considered ethically acceptable. The action's nature insofar as the human subject's basic needs are concerned is not the dominating factor.

The chairperson of the Study Committee on Embryo Research for the United Kingdom (Warnock Report), when defending nontherapeutic research on human embryos, stated: "The argument in effect amounted to this: in a calculation of harms and benefits, the very early embryo need not be counted."[37] The Australian Commission, in rejecting nontherapeutic research on human embryos, stated that no scientific evidence allows a distinction between a "very early embryo" and an "embryo."[38]

Growing Disparity

If the present trends continue, the disparity between the Church's teaching and the study groups' ethical conclusions may grow. Moreover, the clinical practice of some researchers and physicians will veer from traditional ethical theory, such as in some surgeons' willingness to transplant the vital organs of anencephalic infants, thus directly causing their death, to allow others to benefit from their organs.[39]

The disparity raises two questions:

1. Given the history of research involving human beings, does a utilitarian approach to ethical evaluation offer sufficient protection to persons who are subjects in research programs?

2. Could the scientific knowledge sought through nontherapeutic research be acquired without sacrificing human life?

These questions must be answered because the stakes are too great to allow the present disparity of ethical norms to grow wider.

---

1. Vatican Council II, "Pastoral Constitution on the Church in the Modern World," *Gaudium et Spes*, Dec. 7, 1965, no. 35; Pope John Paul II, "The Ethics of Genetic Manipulation," *Origins* 13:23, Nov. 17, 1983, p. 385; Pope Pius XII, "The Foundation of Medical Morality," in *The Human Body: Papal Teachings*, St. Paul Editions, Daughters of St. Paul, Boston, MA, 1960, p. 281; President's Commission for the Study of Ethical Problems in Medicine and Biomedical and Behavior-

al Research, "The Social and Ethical Issues of Genetic Engineering with Human Beings," in *Splicing Life,* U.S. Government Printing Office, Washington, DC, November 1982.

2. Pope Pius XII, "The Intangibility of the Human Person," in *The Human Body,* p. 195; Department of Health, Education, and Welfare, "Ethical Principles and Guidelines for the Protection of Human Subjects of Research," in *The Belmont Report,* U.S. Government Printing Office, Washington, DC, Sept. 30, 1978.

3. Pope Pius XII, "The Intangibility of the Human Person"; President's Commission.

4. President's Commission for the Study of Ethical Problems in Medicine and Biomedical and Behavioral Research, *Protecting Human Subjects,* U.S. Government Printing Office, Washington, DC, March 1981; National Commission for Protection of Human Subjects of Biomedical and Behavioral Research, *Report and Recommendations, Institutional Review Boards,* Department of Health, Education, and Welfare, Washington, DC, 1978.

5. Pope John Paul II.

6. Pope John Paul II; "Ethical Principles and Guidelines for the Protection of Human Subjects of Research"; President's Commission, "The Social and Ethical Issues of Genetic Engineering with Human Beings."

7. Sacred Congregation for the Doctrine of the Faith, "Instruction on Respect for Human Life in Its Origin and on the Dignity of Procreation," *Origins* 16:40, March 19, 1987, pp. 698–711; Pope Pius XII, "The Intangibility of the Human Person"; President's Commission, "The Social and Ethical Issues of Genetic Engineering with Human Beings."

8. Pope Pius XII, "Moral Problems in Medicine," in *The Human Body: Papal Teachings,* p. 311.

9. The Warnock Committee, *Committee of Inquiry into Human Fertilization and Embryology,* Her Majesty's Stationery Office, London, 1984; National Commission for the Protection of Human Subjects of Biomedical and Behavioral Research,

Research on the Fetus, Department of Health, Education, and Welfare, Washington, DC, 1975.

10. Sacred Congregation for the Doctrine of the Faith; *Human Embryo Experimentation in Australia,* Australian Government Publishing Service, Canberra, 1986.

11. Sacred Congregation for the Doctrine of the Faith; Pope Pius XII, "The Intangibility of the Human Person"; President's Commission, "The Social and Ethical Issues of Genetic Engineering with Human Beings."

12. Sacred Congregation for the Doctrine of the Faith; "Ethical Principles and Guidelines for the Protection of Human Subjects of Research."

13. National Commission, *Research on the Fetus.*

14. Pope John Paul II, "Biological Experimentation," *The Pope Speaks,* 28:1, 1983, p. 74; *Human Embryo Experimentation in Australia.*

15. Pope John Paul II, "Church Offers Principles to Guide Medical Advances," *Health Progress,* April 1987, p. 84; U.S. Code of Federal Regulations for Animal Research, Department of Health, Education, and Welfare, Washington, DC, July 25, 1975.

16. Pope Pius XII, "Christian Principles and the Medical Professsion," in *The Human Body: Papal Teachings;* "Ethical Principles and Guidelines for the Protection of Human Subjects of Research."

17. Pope John Paul II, "Church Offers Principles to Guide Medical Advances"; President's Commission, *Protecting Human Subjects.*

18. Pope Pius XII, "Moral Problems in Medicine"; National Commission, *Report and Recommendations, Institutional Review Boards.*

19. Pope John Paul II, "The Ethics of Genetic Manipulation"; President's Commission, *Protecting Human Subjects.*

20. Pope John Paul II, "Biological Experimentation."

21. Pope John Paul II, "The Ethics of Genetic Manipulation."

22. *Committee of Inquiry into Human Fertilization and Embryology;* President's Commission, "The Social and Ethical Issues of Genetic Engineering with Human Beings."

23. *Human Embryo Experimentation in Australia.*
24. National Commission, *Research on the Fetus.*
25. *Committee of Inquiry into Human Fertilization and Embryology.*
26. International Bioethics Summit Conference, "Towards an International Ethic for Research Involving Human Subjects," *IME Bulletin,* May 1987, p. 1.
27. International Bioethics Summit Conference.
28. International Bioethics Summit Conference; *Human Embryo Experimentation in Australia;* President's Commission, "The Social and Ethical Issues of Genetic Engineering with Human Beings."
29. Sacred Congregation for the Doctrine of the Faith; *Human Embryo Experimentation in Australia; Committee of Inquiry into Human Fertilization and Embryology.*
30. Machelle M. Seibel, "A New Era in Reproductive Technology: In Vitro Fertilization, Gamete Intrafallopian Transfer and Donated Gametes and Embryos," *New England Journal of Medicine,* March 31, 1988, pp. 828–834.
31. Sacred Congregation for the Doctrine of the Faith; Pope John Paul II, "The Ethics of Genetic Manipulation."
32. Pope Pius XII, "Christian Principles and the Medical Profession"; Pope Pius XII, "The Intangibility of the Human Person."
33. Pope John Paul II, "Biological Experimentation"; Pope Pius XII, "The Intangibility of the Human Person."
34. "Ethical Principles and Guidelines for the Protection of Human Subjects of Research"; Nuremberg Code, Nuremberg Military Tribunal, *Encyclopedia of Bioethics,* Vol. IV, Free Press, New York, 1946, p. 1764; Medical Research Council of Great Britain, "Responsibility in Investigations on Human Subjects," *Encyclopedia of Bioethics,* Vol. IV, p. 1769.
35. International Bioethics Summit Conference; *Committee of Inquiry into Human Fertilization and Embryology;* President's Commission, "The Social and Ethical Issues of Genetic Engineering with Human Beings."
36. Alisdar MacIntyre, *After Virtue,* University of Notre Dame Press, Notre Dame, IN, 1981.

37. Mary Warnock, "The Warnock Report," *British Medical Journal,* July 10, 1985, p. 187.
38. *Human Embryo Experimentation in Australia.*
39. W. Holzgreve et al., "Kidney Transplantation from Anencephalic Donors," *New England Journal of Medicine,* April 23, 1987, p. 1069.

Healthcare Economics 7

The most common cry in healthcare economics is cost containment. In general, this means that a particular service costs less than it did before or is delivered at the most reasonable price available. The term cost containment is the result of society and the healthcare professions' realization that healthcare costs were climbing at an unacceptable rate and had to be "contained." The mechanism used to do this was to place healthcare in the marketplace and to let the marketplace establish the price. This gave rise to new services, a reexamination of inpatient services to deliver care, and a new prospective payment system.

Some strategies contained the cost of healthcare. Some new structures saved money, but in general the number of dollars spent in healthcare did not decline. With an aging population, the continued development of new technologies, and new health problems, financial costs are not likely to be reduced. The ethical issue is how to live within the confines of available resources.

The assumptions underlying cost containment are that (1) less is better, (2) healthcare institutions are the gatekeepers and controllers of all healthcare costs, (3) healthcare is being delivered at huge profits, and (4) all present and additional services can be delivered at less than the present cost with no change in quantity. Admittedly, there are some examples of this occurring. However, most institutions use their profits to subsidize charity; to reduce debt; to build, replace, and remodel service areas; and to replace and purchase new technologies. Previous reimbursement schemes made this easier than the present prospective payment structures. They also allowed providers to be single-minded in the maximal pursuit of patient benefit. The emphasis on cost containment challenges some of the basic beneficence, autonomy, and social justice values that underlie previous behaviors.

Greater clarity about what cost containment means is needed if new strategies that beneficially reduce some healthcare costs are not to undermine patient care. Doubilet, Weinstein, and McNeil point out that cost effective means many things.[1] It means "cost saving," implying that a less expensive treatment is available. It means "effective care" regardless of cost, with emphasis placed on whether a benefit was obtained. Cost effective means "cost saving" with equal or better outcomes, or it means a therapy is beneficial, more expensive, but worth the extra cost. The authors outline an appropriate use of the term, including the fact that a procedure that costs less but also has some minor health trade-offs can be considered cost effective. The point is that healthcare providers strive for cost-containing measures without clearly specifying what is meant by the term and without making decisions that respect the idiosyncratic needs of patients.

Cost effectiveness needs to bring together two sometimes competing values on a practical level in this discussion. First is the value of sound economics and cost-effective delivery of healthcare. The second is the value of patient benefit and choice. The difficulty is in getting economic structures to have flexibility while still attaining cost-conscious goals. The clue may lie in cost consciousness rather than cost containment.

Prospective pricing for ambulatory surgery and outpatient testing illustrates the point. In a large midwestern city, a 75-year-old woman was brought to the hospital by taxi for outpatient testing for gastrointestinal-related problems. She followed dietary restrictions from the previous night, arrived at the hospital early in the day, and underwent an upper and lower gastrointestinal series, along with blood work and a variety of other tests. As in most outpatient services, meals are not provided and may interfere with the goals of the medical tests. This woman, who lived by herself and who had no family, returned home by taxi. Apparently, sometime in the afternoon, she attempted to make herself something to eat, bent down to pick something up, experienced dizziness, fell, hit her head on the side of a counter or the stove, and suffered a subdural hematoma. She was found on the floor the next morning by a neighbor and was rushed to the hospital for medidal attention. The outpatient service was done to contain costs. Ultimately, it did not.

Two years ago, before prospective payments in diagnosis-related groups, the woman would have been hospitalized overnight, possibly two nights, for these tests. There may be cheaper ways to deliver the same service, such as in an outpatient setting, but circumstances arise when cost may not be the only factor. A significant difference exists between this widowed woman living by herself in her own home and another woman who has others to help, or who by virtue of age or health, is stronger and able to take care of herself.

The value of cost containment is real. The value of outpatient healthcare services for the patient is also significant. In the example, however, overnight accommodations or reimbursed home nursing service may have been necessary and the most cost-conscious choices. Getting the economic structures to bend to these needs seems impossible. Nonetheless, it is a legitimate ethical demand. A lack of financial flexibility for patient benefit can result in patient harm. There is nothing to prevent a more ethical solution if the financial mechanism were more flexible.

The rigidity of the economic structure can be resolved through social and economic principles of cost consciousness meshed with good patient care provided in an appropriate setting. Criteria need to be developed to make this happen. The previous example illustrates the need for economic structures that reflect the human values of healthcare.

Generally, the cost-containing structures of the prospective payment system, preferred provider organizations, and health maintenance organizations, as well as other financing arrangements, raise serious questions about patient benefit becoming a secondary consideration to institutional survival. Also of concern is the maximization of excess revenues over expenses or the goals of efficiency. Physicians and other providers may place institutional, societal, or insurance company needs above the needs of the patient. These priorities are contradictory to the types of values expressed in a more traditional medical model that places the physician-patient relationship at the center of the medical profession. One must be careful not to use the cost-conscious concerns to replace the primary emphasis on patient care.

Medical economics and healthcare ethics are not doomed to contradiction in these settings. Economically, the basic goal is cost-conscious behavior. This is a value. It applies whether one is involved in inpatient or outpatient services. The factors that give rise to increasing costs are not likely to disappear, and benefitting a patient does not mean using every service or all monies available. Cost-conscious behavior must balance economic concerns with patient-centered care.

Conclusion

Today, many are convinced that economic forces should rule the healthcare scene. They believe the marketplace and competition are the forces for reducing healthcare costs and eliminating waste. The model of providing healthcare based on the patient-physician relationship, in which the physician advocated for patients regardless of cost, is a thing of the past. This group further believes that the future for all healthcare rests with economists, business administrators, hospital administrators, and insurance companies. However, these assumptions are questioned by many as the traditional demand for "quality" care and patient satisfaction is perceived.

However, one does not have to choose either healthcare ethics or healthcare economics. The choice is not simple. Economics is one way in which society expresses its preferences and values. Because society values a certain good, such as education, it will support the endeavor with money, often willingly. Society also values its health, but often only at the moment of crisis. Society then expects that healthcare services will be available, effective, and paid for. Public discussion is necessary so that society can decide what it really wants from the healthcare system.

Ethics and economics are not polar opposites. Ethical analysis can help to identify and articulate the values within healthcare that society wants to pursue. Economic structures can then facilitate society's ability to realize them through sound allocation principles and healthy economic structures. Only through sound economic principles can society's health values be attained. Medical ethics and medical economics work in tandem. If they do not, the healthcare of the future will be expensive, but it may not be beneficial.

1. Peter Doubilet, Milton C. Weinstein, and Barbara J. McNeil, "Use and Misuse of the Term 'Cost Effective' in Medicine," *New England Journal of Medicine* 314, Jan. 23, 1986, pp. 253–256.

Patients and Profits: When "The Bottom Line" Dictates Care Levels

8

The economics of today's healthcare marketplace have frayed the once tightly woven fabric of universal patient care. Institutions, no longer so free to underwrite indigent care by shifting costs to paying patients and third-party payors, now find themselves carefully weighing their own fiscal health against their patients' well-being.

All too often, the result is that some of the most vulnerable patients are turned away or receive inadequate care. Take the case of Mrs. Smith, age 81 and widowed, who until her recent two-week hospitalization had lived independently in her own home. During her convalescence, she needs continuing medical care, more than her children can provide either at their homes or hers. Eventually, however, she should be able to resume her previous lifestyle with home healthcare support. The problem is what to do in the interim. Her family thinks Mrs. Smith is being medically short-changed—discharged from the hospital too early because she is a Medicare patient. She cannot afford to cover the cost of interim care herself, and the hospital's social work department has not been able to find her a placement that would address her immediate problems and eventually allow her to return home with limited care.

Or consider the dilemma of Mr. Jones, who needs to have a cataract removed. He is a widower with no family, no close friends, and no church or community contacts to help him following the surgery, which normally is done on an outpatient basis. He offers to pay whatever the hospital charges so that he can spend the night there, but because of Medicare regulations, his request is denied. So far, nobody has been able to help him find an alternative place of care.

And what of the professional staff, who feel squeezed into doing less for greater numbers of patients? Nurses on a medical-surgical floor in a large hospital complain on two fronts: personnel who left have not been replaced, leaving fewer floor nurses available to care for patients; and other supporting services staffs have also been reduced. The nurses say that they are forced to spend less time with their patients and that there is little time to educate family members and patients about their particular conditions. In fact, the nurses charge, quality of care has declined greatly. Although staff reductions are necessary to preserve the hospital's economic viability, the nurses still are beset by frustration, and anger at both the administrators and the physicians sets in.

The Business/Mission Dichotomy

These stories and similar ones follow from both the real and the perceived economic difficulties that mark healthcare today. The stories raise ethical issues that each institution should examine, and they represent problems that healthcare administrators must solve if the institution is to remain viable and quality care delivered.

The subject strikes a note of discord throughout the healthcare community. Virtually the same charges and allegations fly through every institution's rumor mill in times such as these:

- Physicians no longer care enough about patients and their families.
- The administration lacks compassion for the caregivers and will work them until they drop, regardless of the effect on patient care.
- The institution's major concern is to make money rather than to care for the sick.
- Hospitals are natural money-makers and, especially in lean economic times, some of those ever-present profits should be spent on care for the poor.
- Investors in the for-profit sector benefit handsomely at the expense of patients' illnesses. They are willing to provide higher returns to stockholders, increase executive salaries, or build large systems before they will hire more staff or underwrite care for the medically indigent in the institution's home

community.

- Healthcare is just another big business; therefore, its not-for-profit tax status should be denied, hospital profits taxed, and the industry treated as any other.

Some persons argue that institutions effectively have stopped providing charity care and that the situation should be reversed; that is, healthcare facilities should accept all charity patients and provide any and all services that may help them. Others note that the high cost of essential but complex technology sometimes pushes healthcare bills beyond the means of those who once thought themselves adequately insured and financially secure. These persons place the responsibility on federal and state governments to fund indigent and catastrophic healthcare needs.

Obviously, the money to finance care for those who cannot afford to pay must come from somewhere, or medically indigent patients will receive even less care than they do now. But from where? Healthcare administrators quickly point out that unless the costs of indigent care are recouped, healthcare institutions, especially those based among large, indigent populations, eventually would have to shut their doors to all patients. Insurance companies and governments are not necessarily unlimited sources of funding, and they ultimately must answer to their own constituencies for premium and tax increases.

The Financial/Ethical Dichotomy

Whether one examines the individual, tragic stories of the sick person who cannot find adequate healthcare; whether the focus is on the frustrations of the nursing and other allied health professions; or whether the spotlight is directed toward the larger, societal concerns about the general level of charity care delivered in contemporary healthcare facilities, specific but fundamental ethical questions must be answered:

Is healthcare a profession? If so, does its nature imply a certain duty to humankind as well as material reward?

Should a healthcare profession's responsibility to humankind be more strictly applied than that of other professions not responsible for life and death on a daily basis?

Should a healthcare worker's primary concern be to meet the needs of the sick rather than to earn good pay? Should administrators be held to the same standard?

Should healthcare workers and institutions care for all those who are sick and in need? If so, until when?

What happens when revenues no longer cover expenses, and there is not enough money to buy new technology, update physical plants, or pay enough professionals to keep the doors open, let alone provide quality care?

Should healthcare be regarded strictly as a business?

Must healthcare work at maximum efficiency with a top-dollar return on the investments made in it, even if care is denied to all or some who cannot pay?

Or should healthcare be viewed as a hybrid—a mission of universal caring built on a practical, financial base to ensure both its own and society's continuation?

The business/mission dichotomy is one of today's crucial ethical questions. Consensus will not build easily, and the form the answer takes will shape the delivery of healthcare services for decades to come.

How Do Ethics Committees Respond?

Institutional ethics committees (IECs) can address these issues both within committee meetings and through continued education for all personnel. However, this requires careful reflection on the many ethical issues surrounding the extent of society's obligation to deliver needed healthcare services. The IEC's role is advisory and the IEC may not supplant the responsibility or authority of the institution's board of directors or administration, especially in business matters. Although no IEC can be expected to resolve all the fundamental arguments, it can (1) build a consensus within the institution, (2) develop policies that reflect the institution's values concerning treatment of people, including the poor, and (3) help provide a comfort level for professionals in today's difficult economic environment.

First, the IEC should consider its institution's role. Is this institution primarily a business? Is it primarily a moral agent, like a person, with a duty to make promises and follow through on commitments to the community in which it exists? If there is a dual role, which one is subordinate, and to what extent?

The Business Role

If an institution's primary role is as a business, then its value commitments should express the intention to maximize the return on investments made by individuals or the community. Economies of scale must be a priority. Attempts must be made to deliver the best possible care with the least number of people. The paying patients and their immediate medical needs must receive the greatest attention, with less consideration to issues (e.g., indigent care) perceived as technically not the institution's responsibility. The bottom-line value may be to make money in order to continue the institution's existence. In general, these values will be realized through a focus on profitability, sophisticated studies of consumer satisfaction, and appropriate community relations conveying that the institution is sound and ready to serve those who can afford healthcare. Business-focused values do not preclude the institution from providing some charitable work, but they guide most efforts toward services that are predominantly profitable and/or reimbursed by insurance companies. Services that require great expenditures with little likelihood of recouping the investment probably will not be offered. Because some services, such as emergency room care, may be misused or attract those who cannot afford healthcare, they may be offered only during certain hours or not at all.

Role of Moral Agent

If the institution's primary role is that of a moral agent, it must be viewed as a person able to make commitments based on conscious responses to those in need. Further, its promises must be evaluated as a person's promises would be: Does the institution, in fact, live up to the promises it has made?

If an institution commits to caring for health needs that cannot or will not be met elsewhere in the community, it creates an expectation that it exists to provide service. This expectation can lead to institution-threatening financial difficulties, however, if a certain percentage of patients cannot pay for their care. The institution must be able to generate some sort of excess revenue over expenses to meet the obligations that its promise requires. This points to the need for community support, since the healthcare relationship is between both the institution and the people for whom it cares.

An institution's commitment to care for its community also must include other, implicit promises. These include (1) to provide the best possible care, measured through a quality assurance committee seeking to ensure that competent, capable professionals care for the needs of the institution's patients, and (2) to evaluate regularly the healthcare facility's growth and allocation of resources. Technological acquisitions and other major expenditures should be measured by their potential to help the institution meet a wide variety of needs. The purchase of an expensive, specialized piece of technology, for example, may benefit only a few patients. The institution must decide whether to forego the purchase in favor of another piece of equipment that may have wider application.

Hybridizing Healthcare's Roles

Regardless of an institution's primary role, arguments must be made for its profitability or recovery of costs. Even the best-intentioned care cannot be delivered if an institution cannot pay its own bills over the long term. So the question is not, "Must money be made?" but, "Who gains from the money that is made?" Will the beneficiary be the community at large, and the medically indigent in particular? Or will the excess money be returned to stockholders who made the initial investment in the institution?

Even for-profit institutions will not be reimbursed for all services they provide. So how will the cost of those services be recovered? If the institutional role is primarily that of a business, a priority may be to do away with services that are not reimbursed. If the main role is one of moral agent, then ways must be found to provide for the tangential needs that arise out of illness.

A place in the budget must be made to provide for social services, pastoral care, and the comfort and support of family members. Whether healthcare facilities are run as businesses or as moral agents, all institutions must cover the costs of providing services, updating technology and facilities, adequately compensating the employees, and responding in some degree to community need.

Few patients can pay for all their healthcare costs themselves. As a result, people seek insurance, government, or other assistance to help pay for their care. Until fairly recently, these third-party payers helped healthcare institutions remain viable through cost shifting, or paying more than the actual cost of a covered patient's care to help make up the losses generated by charity care. That changed when third-party payers decided that the costs charged to them exceeded what they were willing to pay. The result of these financial pressures has been the move toward healthcare cost containment and the development of a variety of payment plans that may or may not reflect the values that vulnerable people have when they are ill. In addition, the requirements imposed by the reimbursement mechanisms affect the way that healthcare institutions deliver their services.

Examining Values and Financial Concerns

Ethics committees should ask themselves what values are reflected in the financial concerns faced by their institution. One value might be how the institution structures programs to provide charity care in an era of cost containment. Today's managed care programs, alternative delivery systems, discounts, and contractual allowances establish very tight financial constraints under which the institution must work to make ends meet at the end of a fiscal year. In general, these programs and allowances reimburse the institution on a fair-cost basis, without cost shifting for services delivered to medically indigent patients. The extent to which an institution enters into such restrictive contracts reflects one aspect of its commitment to overall services. Cost shifting may be an unpopular method of caring for charity patients, but unless the bulk of society helps carry the load, institutions will be forced to find other ways to cover the costs of charity care. Those "other ways" say something about the institution's values.

Within the institution, greater emphasis on financial management results, when possible, in predetermining a prospective patient's ability to pay. Before admission, the patient usually is asked for proof of insurance or other means of payment. There has been an increase in the use of consumer credit cards and other credit arrangements as families personally shoulder the financial burden of healthcare as far as their credit limits will permit. Hospitals hire bill collectors to follow up on outstanding accounts and to identify cases of charity care vs. bad debt so that as much revenue as possible can be collected without tarnishing the institution's caring image. Again, how the financial management structures are established reflects the institution's fundamental values.

Healthcare facilities also try to take advantage of economies of scale to cut costs while attracting more consumers to their services. The development of group purchasing arrangements, multiinstitutional healthcare systems, pricing strategies, and horizontal and vertical integration can help to cut waste while reflecting basic values. For example, an institution may save money by entering into a group purchasing agreement that permits it to buy certain equipment at a discount. However, the charity question returns when, even if the reduced costs are passed along, some needy patients cannot pay for use of the equipment.

Moving Toward Solutions

Examining the economics of healthcare can be a daunting prospect to IEC members unskilled in the finer points of industry finance. Finding an appropriate channel through which to ask questions and interpret answers is the first, often most difficult step. Once begun, questions about the dominant values expressed by the institution through its business, professional, and fiscal policies will begin to flow.

First, IECs can look into the value of money, otherwise

known as profits or cost recovery, to the institution. On the positive side, proper cash flow is necessary for any institution to survive, regardless of whether its status is as an investor-owned, for-profit, not-for-profit, community, or religiously affiliated facility. On the negative side, preoccupation with profitability can have a devastating effect on many patients' access to services and on the opportunity for families to participate in the healing experience.

Ethics committees also can address some fiscal concerns by examining the underlying values and costs of some medical interventions. For instance, if the institution has clear policies on how to deal with death and dying, it often can avoid spending great amounts of money to sustain inappropriately the physical existence of a patient who should be allowed to die. Organ transplants and other services that may or may not benefit patients also should be examined in a similar light.

Second, as healthcare centers seek horizontal and vertical integration—control of factors that lead a patient into an institution and care for the patient after discharge—primary values of care, family, and personal choice become paramount.

Third, IECs must look at the implied value of an institution's commitment to care from both the narrow and the broad perspectives. Does healthcare include an integrated set of services designed to address the needs of the whole person, or is the focus solely on physiological and psychological medical intervention for particular diseases? The ever-present problem —how to pay for services that do not necessarily address the patient's immediate physiological and psychological needs— arises again. If an institution broadly defines health and health services, alternatives may be developed to maximize the health benefits to patients while attending to costs in an economically sound way. The difference is between whether the focus begins with the *mission* perspective and then finds ways to finance it, or whether *business* and finances basically drive the institution.

Beyond Individual Institutions

One reason IECs sometimes encounter difficulty dealing with these ethical issues is because the solutions are more encompassing than any single institution or system. The health-care community must work as a whole to bring these matters to society's attention and thus effect change. The business community has been successful in pointing to the high cost of healthcare benefits and its impact on the cost of consumer goods.

Society now must recognize that healthcare is an expensive proposition, especially considering the constant evolution of technology and the legitimate value of the promotion of life. This is particularly clear in cases of premature or ill neonates, serious trauma, stroke, heart disease, organ transplantation, cancer, and AIDS. These patients may benefit significantly from expensive medical interventions. What will be the basis for deciding whether they are allowed to try?

The real costs of services must be identified by those who understand the wide parameters of care essential to help a patient through an illness. If the voices of the business or governmental communities are the only ones raised on these issues, no one in the healthcare field should be surprised to face ever-increasing pressure to do more with less. Unless healthcare centers and the organizations that represent them personally, professionally, and institutionally try to work with business and with local, state, and federal governments, only the people with the greatest financial interest will make decisions. And those decisions may not necessarily be in the best interest of either institutions or patients.

There is a need for serious and long-term debate about both the macroallocation of dollars in healthcare and the microallocation of an institution's resources for the people it serves. Most analysts of the healthcare environment suggest that regional rather than individual solutions are necessary. This requires that institutions and their personnel in all disciplines, whether physicians, nurses, technicians, administrators, or others, clearly understand their own values and commitments before they begin the necessary dialogue with other facilities and organizations in the region.

Discussions can be moved forward by the IEC as it examines both the basic values that underlie care within the institution and the implications of those values as expressed by institutional policies and delivery of service. The use of technology should be discussed; specifically, how technology reflects values and how it can best be used given the institution's particular resources. Whether the discussion encompasses technology or the work of individual fields of healthcare, the same questions eventually must be raised and answered in public forums.

In addition, discussion must continue about the value of proprietary-owned and non-proprietary-owned healthcare centers. Questions addressing financial concerns, perception of need, and the desire for adequate, efficient, and effective healthcare should be covered.

Ethics committees also can extend their research and influence by beginning to respond to the growing public policy issues on local, state, and national levels. Already ripe for discussion are (1) changes in Medicare and Medicaid reimbursement; (2) expansion of Medicaid services, as suggested in many states; (3) rules and regulations that govern nursing homes and affect hospitals; and (4) financial reimbursement plans.

Specific expertise is essential, however, to address public policy concerns credibly. Depending on its makeup, structure, and time constraints, an IEC may not be appropriate to serve as the catalyst for public debate. At the minimum, however, the committee should articulate institutional values to the public. This requires that IEC members learn about the complex network of finances, reimbursement, and costs of medical care. It may take months of study and deliberation, but the worthwhile result will be clarifying and carrying out the institution's fundamental values.

Conclusion

When an ethics committee examines the most basic values underlying its institution's philosophy of patient care, it does so looking to the future of healthcare. The IEC is the primary testing ground and must be able to lead an educated and informed discussion of the business/mission dichotomy not just within the institution, but throughout the community. A forum that includes many people from many fields of the healthcare industry will help clearly establish healthcare's underlying values, the ways in which it finances those values, and the impact its decisions have on patients, families, the institution, the community, and society.

Investor-Owned Healthcare Corporations: Are They Ethical?   9

Does the type of institutional ownership present an ethical issue when healthcare is concerned? In other words, is there anything about healthcare which would lead one to say that healthcare would be better offered by a not-for-profit corporation rather than by an investor-owned for-profit corporation?* The presence of for-profit or investor-owned corporations in healthcare is well established, and their activities have been evaluated frequently in relation to not-for-profit corporations. Most of these evaluations have all been made from an economic perspective.[1]

This evaluation of for-profit healthcare corporations will be from an ethical perspective. Ethics is the science and art of making beneficial human decisions, decisions that help individuals fulfill their innate and cultural needs. If one has a need, then fulfilling that need is a good or value for the person concerned. Thus, ethics is concerned with needs, goods, and values. Values influence and determine human actions and human personality.[2] When a person has a need and capacity to pursue a value, we say that person has a *right*. If the need is innate or intrinsic to the person's well-being or goal in life, the right to which the need gives rise is called *fundamental* or *inalienable*. Rights are fostered, protected, and attained through responsible actions. Thus, our consideration of values necessarily brings into discussion the rights and responsibilities of those who need healthcare and those who provide this care.

In this study, therefore, we are concerned with the human values intrinsic to or intimately associated with striving for health and the provisions of healthcare. After delineating and explaining these values, we consider whether or not investor-owned healthcare corporations promote or present the acquisi-

*The terms *investor-owned* and *for-profit* are often used synonymously. For our purposes in this study, it is more accurate to use the term *investor-owned*. (See p. 67.)

tion of such values. The discussion is divided into two parts. In the first we consider healthcare and the values, rights, responsibilities of people and corporations who offer healthcare. In the second section we discuss the theory and motives of investor-owned for-profit healthcare corporations in order to evaluate their conformity to the values, rights, and responsibilities treated in the first part.

Observers of the medical care scene in the United States may react to the consideration of values in healthcare with skepticism at best. Most Americans in business and administrators are loathe to talk or write about values.[3] Those who do pay lip service to values tend to treat them as gross abstractions, acceptable for discussion at conventions but too impractical to apply when discussing planning or operations. Moreover, many would say that applying value considerations to the present healthcare situation in the United States is anachronistic. After all, since investor-owned corporations are part of the healthcare scene in the United States, what is the point of calling into question their right to exist?

From the outset, we wish to declare that we have no illusions about the healthcare milieu in the United States. Although the quality of U.S. healthcare is defensible, the delivery system is flawed, thus, many people do not have sufficient access to healthcare. The inequities of care, shortcomings in funding, monopolistic tendencies of suppliers, and lack of access for the poor have been too thoroughly documented to allow anyone to defend the present system of delivery (or lack of system) as an ideal.[4]

In response to those who react skeptically to this value analysis, we would offer two considerations. First, by no stretch of the imagination could the provision of healthcare in the United States be put forward as the ideal. If change and renewal in the provision of healthcare is needed, then beneficial changes will not result if we merely tamper with the present delivery methods. Rather, let the changes in the system be dramatic, fundamental, and oriented to achieving the values inherent in healthcare. If we contend, therefore, that the breakdown in the provision of the U.S. healthcare system is caused by a substitution of money instead of service as the goal of healthcare, it is not sufficient to say "the service model of healthcare no longer exists in this country." Rather, if the service model responds to the needs and rights of the people seeking healthcare, we must ask, "What changes are needed in the attitudes, ethics, and laws of people and corporations offering healthcare in order to restore the service model?"

Second, in response to the view that a value-oriented analysis of healthcare is overly idealistic, especially in face of present realities, we would affirm the fundamental worth and importance of value orientation. As Peters and Waterman state:

> Let us suppose that we were asked for one all-purpose bit of advice for management, one truth that we were able to distill from the excellent companies we researched. We might be tempted to reply, 'Figure out your value system. Decide what your company stands for. What does your enterprise do that gives everyone the most pride? Put yourself out ten or twenty years in the future; what would you look back on with greatest satisfaction?'[5]

With these caveats in mind, let us proceed to consider the values inherent in healthcare and the rights and responsibilities associated with the attainment of those values.

Meaning of Healthcare

Health and healthcare are interdependent. Restoring health and preventing illness (a lack of health) are the goals of healthcare; thus, to understand the values associated with healthcare, one must possess a clear idea of human health. Ask the physician, nurse, or hospital administrator, "What is health?" and you are likely to receive a blank look in reply. Although thousands of people are involved in healthcare in the United States, no consensus exists concerning the nature of health. In an effort to formulate a health planning guide, Henrik

Blum suggests the following definition:

> Health consists of the capacity of an organism (1) to maintain a balance appropriate to its age and social needs, in which it is reasonably free of gross dissatisfaction, discomfort, disease, or disability; and (2) to behave in ways which promote the survival of the species as well as the self-fulfillment or enjoyment of the individual.[6]

Blum ends his discussion of human health with the brief formula, "Health is the state of being in which an individual does the best with the capacities he has, and acts in ways that maximize his capacities."[7] Because a human being is an organism, it is an open system. In maintaining balance or homeostasis, therefore, persons are continually relating to their environment. For our purposes, then, we conceive of health as optimal human functioning, which implies not only an internal harmony and consistency of function, but also the capacity of the person to maintain oneself in the environment.

To understand more fully this notion of health, one must understand the needs and functions of the human person and how these are related. Otherwise, one has a confused notion of human health. Briefly, human beings are born with the capacity to perform certain functions in response to felt needs. They have a capacity for knowledge, and because they feel a need for truth in order to understand and fulfill their purpose in life, they perform the function of learning. It is widely acknowledged that there are four categories of human needs and corresponding functions:

1. *Biological or physiological functions* correspond to needs human beings share with all living organisms: to maintain themselves homeostatically in a dynamic relation with their environment, to grow and mature to full biological development, and to continue the species through reproduction. Biologically, persons need food, air, shelter, warmth, and so on.

2. *Psychological functions* correspond to the human needs

to sense, imagine, and feel. These enable persons to meet their needs for security, affirmation, and acceptance.

3. *Social functions* enable individuals to meet their needs for self-control and for peaceful and productive social relations within the context of their culture.

4. *Spiritual or creative functions* enable people to fulfill their need for commitment, integration, and transcendence. This function enables persons not only to live within a culture, but to criticize it, transcend it, and contribute to it.

Limits of Medical Care

Given these basic needs and functions, it is extremely important to discern how they are related, since this will provide a blueprint for the quest for health and the limits of medical care. Is one function more important than another? If so, will it contribute more to health? Are the relationships among the various functions cooperative or competitive? Can one need or function be sacrificed for another without impairing the individual's health?

These four functions are not stories in a building, one on top of the other, but rather interrelated dimensions of human activity. Just as the length, height, and depth of a cube can be distinguished conceptually for sake of study, but not separated in reality, so the four functions of the human act are interconnected. Every truly human act involves all four functions. A human spiritual act, whether it be the creative act of a scientist or the loving act of a parent, at the same time involves a biological, psychological, and social function. True, one type of function will predominate in a human act, but all types will be present. The task of the creative function is to integrate the biological, psychological, and social functions. Thus, creative functions are the deepest, most central, and most complete. At the same time, however, all these activities are rooted in and dependent on the other functions in a network of interrelations. One cannot think unless one's brain is physiologically sound. Moreover, each function is to a certain extent autonomous, structurally and functionally differentiated, so that when help is needed to restore function, each function is served by a different discipline. To restore the physiological function, one trained in medicine is called; for the psychological function, one trained in psychology or psychiatry; for the social function, a social counselor or lawyer; for the creative-spiritual function, a teacher or spiritual director.

Value of the Person

No matter which type of professional is called on in an effort to integrate or improve human function—that is, to restore or maintain health—that individual does not assume the right to make decisions for the person in question. The professional must always be cognizant of the interrelatedness of all human functions, even if his or her effort is directed toward restoring only one function. Thus, the creative function of making free, value-based decisions is retained by the person in question. This creative decision-making function is generally considered the essence of human worth and the primary activity by which one fulfills one's destiny or purpose in life. Through that type of creative action basic decisions and commitments are made that lead to the integration of all human functions. By virtue of this function or power, people are of inestimable worth, and anyone who seeks to help another regain health must do so with reverence for this worth. The reverence and respect for the person and for the creative function are the basis for requiring informed consent and other ethical norms, such as confidentiality and truth telling, that have been stressed in the practice of medicine in recent years.

Meaning and Values of Medical Care

From the previous consideration of human health and human function, it is clear that physicians and all other medical care professionals must be concerned primarily with healing and physiological and psychological functions. However, their efforts at restoring these functions or preventing their failure must be performed with the awareness of the interrelatedness of all human functions. Thus, the term *healthcare* is more comprehensive than the term medical care because it refers to the restoration of the individual's capacity for integrative functioning. Medical care refers more properly to what physicians and nurses do to help people regain or maintain health, that is, to restore physiological and psychological functioning. Confusion about the appropriate domain of medical care can lead to serious mistakes in the physician-patient relationship or in utilizing the resources of society. Physicians who do not realize the interrelatedness of all human functions might think they have the right to make all decisions for the patient; health planning might be directed only to the amelioration of physiological problems without regard for their origin in psychological, social, or spiritual problems.

In keeping with the notion of human health that we have offered, the patient is not passive in medical care. Rather, he or she retains the right of choosing medical means in accord with his or her value system. Even though patients present themselves in a wounded state of health, as a result of which they have lost some degree of self-determination, patients' power to make their own decisions must be respected by the physician and all other persons in healthcare. Because of the good in question, and because a need exists to respect the spiritual integrity of the person who comes for help, *a specific type of relationship arises between the physician and the patient,* known familiarly as the professional relationship. The heart of this relationship is the avowal (profession) on the part of one person that he or she is willing to help another person attain a very important human good while at the same time respecting his or her personal worth and dignity. The professional promises *to serve* people in need, the ability of the person to pay for the help being a secondary consideration.

Today the term *professional* is applied casually to anyone who is adept at a job or trade and seeks to perform his or her work in a competent and honest manner. Thus, we might call an accountant or a plumber a professional. In the proper meaning of the term, however, to be a professional implies something more than knowledge and skill. It implies as well a desire and ability to help a person with impaired function so that the person can become a better human being. Although an accountant or plumber may help a person with his or her income tax or water supply, those services do not necessarily make the recipient a better human being. What makes a person a better human being is the restoration of the capacity for fully integrated functioning, which in turn enables the person to strive for a meaningful life in an effective manner.

The professional, then, is concerned with a good that enables the person to become a better human being. Robert Merton explains the values of a professional as follows: "First, the value placed upon systematic knowledge and intellect: knowing. Second, the value placed upon mechanical skill and trained capacity: doing. And third, the value placed upon putting this conjoint knowledge and skill to work in the service of others: helping."[8]

Kenneth Underwood further explains the service dimension of public responsiblity: "These four concerns—concern for persons, trained skills, values and basic theory, and public responsiblity—are the central themes of professional ideology always mentioned in the sociological literature on the professions and the professions' statement of purpose."[9]

Given the service value in the relationship between the professional and the human person in need of help, it is evident that the relationship must be built on trust. This is especially true in medicine, where the patient's vulnerability is multidimensional and the patient-physician relationship is intrinsically imbalanced. As Pellegrino and Thomasma state: "Medicine is . . . assistance and explanation, skill and commitment, all based on an ethic of trust which, in turn, is based on the ontological and sociological reality of an imbalanced relationship."[10]

To develop trust in the patient, the medical professional must do four things:

1. Develop knowledge and skill in medicine, good judgment, and facility at performing procedures. Personal warmth does not substitute for medical expertise.

2. Show concern for the patient's well-being. Trust will never exist if the patient believes that the physician is concerned only about the fee or is acting out of mere routine as a machine

or a functionary of a for-profit enterprise. Thus, the professional undertakes to help the client not because the client is worthy of help, nor because he or she is able to pay for the service, but primarily because of human need and the essential human rights based on need rather than on merit or ability to pay.

3. Communicate effectively with patients. A well-known study of hospital care showed that a high percentage of patients were incorrectly diagnosed because of the failure of physicians to listen carefully to patients' complaints and to recognize nonmedical factors in their condition.

4. Set or refuse an appropriate fee. Nothing destroys a trust relationship more quickly and more thoroughly than emphasis on money as the basis for the relationship. Medical professionals, because of the good involved and the relationship to the patient, should not be paid according to laws of supply and demand. The good they are concerned with, namely, health and life, is beyond price. At no time in the history of medicine has the profession operated totally in accordance with the market system, because there have always been people who needed help desperately but could not pay for it. Either the professional had to offer service free to the poor, or a third party, such as a religious institution or the state, had to pay for it.

If our account of the values inherent in the medical relationship is accurate, then it is clear why profit cannot be the primary basis of any profession, and why it must be considered a secondary and highly variable feature. Traditionally, a principle fundamental to all professions has been that the professional must be ready to give services free to those who are *in need* but cannot pay. The medical profession, as with any true profession, must rest not on bargaining or supply and demand, but on trust and service to those in need. No monetary value can be set on the spirtitual guidance given by a minister, the defense of human rights provided by a lawyer, or the search for truth shared by a teacher. Nor can any price be set on the services of a physician in the battle to live. Thus, professional fees are not payments measured by the value of the service provided, which is truly priceless. Rather, they are a stipend that should be based solely on what professionals require to live in a manner that will free them to work without distraction, with liberty of mind and health of body, and to fulfill adequately present and future family and social obligations. That some physicians still recognize this professional tenet is clear from a recent statement of a prominent physician: "We must also be reasonable in our own demands for recompense. Doctors deserve a good living, but not an extravagant one. Greed and medical care are not compatible."[11]

Ultimately, the rewards in any profession are not to be found in extraneous gain. The rewards are intrinsic: the satisfaction of knowledge and of interesting and absorbing work and the joy that comes from helping people in their striving for a better life and from serving the individual and common good. Such an altruistic ideal is not easy to realize, nor is it often realized in its purest form; but even when imperfectly realized, it is the source of the medical profession's purpose and values. Whether this ideal is explicit or implicit in the physician's practice, for centuries medicine has brought out the best in people because of this ideal.

The specific responsibilities associated with professional responsiblity fostering trust apply as much to healthcare corporations such as clinics, hospitals, or surgicenters as to individual healthcare professionals. Corporations are recognized by law as entities (moral persons) pursuing the same goals as individuals, although ostensibly in a more effective manner. Thus, the healthcare corporation is assessed and its responsiblities determined not on the basis of its material constitution, since this differs from that of the individual person, but on the basis of its purpose. Corporations in the field of medical care, therefore, must have the same primary goal as healthcare professionals: service to individuals in need of healing.

To build an atmosphere of trust, the corporation must maintain fiscal stability and make a surplus or profit. The ethical health corporation does not use its surplus to enrich investors, however, because this makes profit rather than service the purpose of the healthcare endeavor. Those who object that they can make a profit for investors and strive for service-oriented, compassionate medical care at the same time are confusing contradictory objectives. The situation in healthcare in the

United States illustrates this dichotomy. More and more, the poor are underserved as profit becomes the overriding goal of healthcare corporations. Unfortunately, even some not-for-profit healthcare corporations misplace their priorities. Moreover, taking money out of the medical care system makes it more expensive than it should be and often results in more affluent individuals profiting from the suffering of the less affluent.

Resulting Value Statements

In view of this analysis of healthcare and the professional-patient relationship, the following value statements are normative for individuals and corporations involved in healthcare:

1. The primary and overriding purpose of medical care must be a desire to serve all whose physiological or psychological health is impaired in order to enable them to lead a better life. Thus, ensuring access to medical care for all persons is an important value to all healthcare professionals.

2. Those offering medical care must remember and respect the worth and autonomy of the individual.

3. The patient-physician relationship must be permeated by trust.

4. Medical care should not be considered a commodity, something to be bought or sold in a market system. This is because medical care is a precious and vital good to which no price can be attached, and because it is a prerequisite to the attainment of other human goods as well as to the pursuit of a meaningful life. Moreover, those who are most in need of medical care often have the least ability to pay for it.

5. Surplus funds over and above the money needed for expenses should not be taken out of the healthcare system by distribution to individual investors. Rather, the only appropriate disposition of any surplus is to continue and improve the quality of and the access to medical care.

6. Although persons and corporations offering medical care should receive an adequate stipend for service, they must fulfill their fundamental responsiblity to care for those who cannot offer a stipend.

7. Because of their skill and their prominence in society,

medical care professionals and corporations must assume leadership in the effort to establish equity of access to medical care.

Investor-Owned Medical Care Corporations

In this section, after presenting a working definition of the investor-owned healthcare corporation, we offer an ethical evaluation of these corporations in light of the value statments for healthcare professionals and corporations developed in the previous section.

Nature of Investor-Owned Corporations

The term *investor-owned medical care corporation* refers to a for-profit corporation, usually a hospital or long term care facility, that offers medical care to patients and:

1. Involves a market system approach to healthcare, treating it basically as a commodity

2. Makes a profit for investors who are not personally involved in offering healthcare

3. Considers, usually in self-description, "making a profit" to be the primary goal of the enterprise

4. Renounces the personal responsibility of the corporation to care for the poor and to develop equitable access to healthcare for all persons

Clearly, the goals and actions of the investor-owned medical care corporations do not correspond to the value statements developed in the previous section. Neither the goals nor the the activities of these corporations coincide with service-oriented, compassionate medical care. Moreover, these corporations consider medical care to be not a profession, but a business—or, as the currently popular, misguided phrase has it, "an industry." These corporations take money out of the medical care system and refuse to assume the responsibility of offering care for the poor and developing equal access to healthcare.

To substantiate our position that the description of investor-owned medical care corporations just offered is accurate, and that these corporations are unethical because they do not serve the proper values of medical care, we consider the arguments often put forth in support of investor-owned medical care corporations. The main defenses for the existence of these corporations state that (1) treating medical care as a commodity will improve the system of delivery by lowering costs and making the system more efficient and more effective, (2) the investor-owned hospitals pay taxes and thus help care for the poor, and (3) all medical care corporations must make a profit. Therefore, no difference exists between charitable and investor-owned hospitals.[12]

Medical Care as Commodity

Proponents of investor-owned hospitals state that treating healthcare as a commodity is a logical step in creating a more effective and cost-efficient healthcare system. Competition is put forward as the solution to healthcare expense. Competition has led to higher prices in healthcare, however, especially given the well-documented realization that competition as we know it in U.S. healthcare is a word more than a reality.[13] Although cost efficiency is a worthwhile goal, it must be subordinated to the more important and fundamental goal of ensuring equitable access to medical care. Thus, to consider the assertion about effectiveness and efficiency from a value perspective, the type of good offered in healthcare must be considered carefully.

In its report entitled *Securing Access to Health Care,* the President's Commission for the Study of Ethical Problems in Medicine and Biomedical and Behavioral Research points out the nature of the human good involved in healthcare and the essential immorality of the market approach to healthcare:

> The private market does not adjust the financial burden of care to differences in income. Yet poverty and ill health are correlated—with the causal factors working in both directions. Therefore, the poor are in a double bind; they need more medical care but they have less money to purchase it or less insurance to secure it.[14]

Thus, the market approach deprives those persons of

healthcare who need it most. With many cultural needs, it is appropriate to expect people to adjust their desires and wants (the fulfillment of their potential) to their ability to pay. The person who desires to see a movie or buy an automobile must pay for it. In this manner, other people are enabled to earn income and purchase goods and services.

Healthcare differs from most other goods and services, however, because it is a good on which the acquisition of income is based and on which most other goods depend. It is an innate need. If one is ill or infirm, it is difficult to earn money to pay for the care that will enable one to regain health. Often the illness or infirmity is so severe that maintaining a limited health status is all that can be foreseen. Are people of such limited capacity to be declared ineligible for healthcare because they cannot pay for it? Health, insofar as it is the absence of pain, suffering, or serious disability, is what has been called a *primary* or *innate* need. That is, despite any other goals or preferences a person might have, it is clear that health is good for that individual. As the economist Eli Ginzburg points out, "To view the practice of medicine as just another business undertaking like retailing or banking is to be blind to the role of agency in the work of a professional."[15]

We should no more look on medical care as a market commodity than we should police and fire protection. An element of public good and dire need exists in both these services, as in healthcare, which makes it unethical to demand payment from those unable to pay. Thus, cost effectiveness is only one dimension—and a secondary one—of effectiveness in medical care. The primary measure is the service relationship and the access to care afforded to those who are most in need.

Taxes and Care for the Poor

Although we endorse a professional-patient relationship that involves a professional's personal responsibility to care for the poor, this does not signify that responsibility for improving the provision of healthcare rests solely with the healthcare professional or with healthcare corporations. Ensuring access to healthcare is an obligation that must be borne by all the people and institutions that make up the society.[16] Although state and federal governments are elements in society, they do not remove the personal responsiblity from individuals or institutions. Therefore, it is invalid for physicians, nurses, hospitals, or other healthcare corporations to say, "Let the federal government take care of the poor." Nor is it valid to say, "We pay taxes, and care for the poor should come out of our taxes." Medical professionals, whether individuals or corporations, must realize their personal ethical responsibility to help those who cannot help themselves. They will fulfill this responsibility through personal care and through political activity designed to help those in need. The President's Commission expressed the complex balance of personal and social responsiblities in the following manner:

> Society has a moral obligation to ensure that everyone has access to adequate care without being subject to excessive burdens . . . But the recognition of a collective or societal obligation does not imply that government should be the only or even the primary institution involved in the complex enterprise of making healthcare available. It is the Commission's view that the societal obligation to ensure equitable access for everyone may best be fulfilled in this country by a pluralistic approach that relies upon the coordinated contributions of actions by both the private and public sectors . . . There is a strong tradition of private charity in the United States, including free services by health professionals, and charitable organizations continue to play an important role in healthcare delivery.[17]

Every person and corporation involved in healthcare has an ethical obligation to care for the poor, individually and collectively, and to work for equitable access to the system. The government should move in as required to fill the gaps and ensure equity of access. Do investor-owned healthcare corporations accept a personal responsibility? Paul Starr notes:

> The profit-making hospitals clearly benefit from the structure of private health insurance and can be counted on to oppose any national health program that might threaten to end private reimbursement. The corporate health services industry will also represent a powerful new force resisting public accountability and participation. A corporate sector in healthcare is also likely to aggravate inequalities in access to healthcare. Profit-making enterprises are not interested in treating those who cannot pay. The voluntary hospital may not treat the poor the same as the rich, but they do treat them and often treat them well.[18]

The de facto behavior of investor-owned healthcare corporations seems to confirm our evaluation. Leaders of the investor-owned hospitals have been heard to deny a personal responsibility to care for the poor. Michael Bromberg of the Federation of American Hospitals stated that investor-owned hospitals pay taxes, "which in turn are used to support public hospitals."[19] One doubts that the accountants preparing the tax returns for investor-owned hospitals are told, "Don't cut any corners or claim any borderline exemptions; remember, our taxes will mean better healthcare for the poor." It seems far more likely that efforts would be made to pay as little tax as possible so there will be more profits to enrich investors. In other words, one seeks evidence to substantiate Bromberg's inference that investor-owned hospitals are committed to their responsibility to support the efforts of society to provide adequate access to healthcare. For healthcare professionals and corporations, care for the poor is both a personal and a social responsibility. Is there evidence that either responsibility is fulfilled in investor-owned medical care? The pertinent literature does not justify an affirmative response.[20]

Profit and Medical Care

Could it not be argued that making a surplus or a profit is incumbent on all healthcare corporations if they are to continue in existence, and that therefore investor-owned corporations have a place in healthcare? Here we must be careful in our understanding of terms. A profit simply means that a corporate entity takes in more than it spends. In this sense, every healthcare corporation must make a profit to care for the future as well as the present. If there is no profit, the corporation will cease to exist. The denominations "for-profit" and "not-for-profit," therefore, are not clear enough to be significant in this discussion. Rather, the concern is what *happens* to the profits. Returning them to the healthcare system by using the surplus to improve quality of care, improve access, or provide needed equipment or buildings is an ethical use of profits; distributing them to investors who have no direct interest in supplying medical care is not.[21] To distribute profits to investors has two results, both of which are unethical: (1) money is removed from the healthcare system, thus making healthcare cost more than it should; and (2) the trust that should characterize medicine is weakened and eventually destroyed. Paul Starr points out the inevitability of these results when discussing the consequences of the "coming of the corporation" into medical care:

> The organizational culture of medicine used to be dominated by the ideals of professionalism and voluntarism, which softened the underlying acquisitive activity. The restraint exercised by those ideals now grows weaker. The "health center" of one era is the "profit center" of the next.[22]

Not only do investor-owned medical corporations take money out of the system, but the manner in which they obtain their profits is open to ethical questions. "Creaming" the lucrative services and patients and avoiding unprofitable activities, which are part of a complete medical care service, is not uncommon for investor-owned corporations.[23] "Dumping" is another typical practice today.[24] In the process of "creaming and dumping," the goal of compassionate service to ailing humanity is supplanted by the goal of profit. Is it possible to take surplus funds out of the system and still have service as the primary goal of medical care? Long ago a wise man said, "No one can serve two masters." Today the true goal of the investor-owned hospital is clearly evidenced in the following vignette:

> To stimulate admissions, Humana offers physicians office space at a discount in buildings next to its hospitals and even guarantees first-year incomes of $60,000. It then keeps track of the revenues each doctor generates. "They let you know if you're not keeping up to expectations," says one young physician. Humana's president is frank about what happens if they fail to produce: "I'm damn sure I'm not going to renegotiate their office leases. They can practice elsewhere."[25]

Conclusion

Because of the values inherent in healthcare and in the pursuit of health, and because of the values, dispositions, and attitudes that should typify the individuals and corporations that offer healthcare in the United States, it seems that investor-owned healthcare corporations are unethical. They neither strive for nor reflect the values proper to healthcare. In fact, the conditions and attitudes that allow investor-owned healthcare corporations to survive in our society lead us to ask some far more serious questions:
- What type of society are we creating for ourselves?
- What type of society are we creating for future generations?
- What values do we wish to dominate society in the present and in the future?
- Are we espousing values that promote service, trust, and

compassion for the weak, or values that promote competition, exploitation, and profits for the strong at the expense of the weak?

There are some goods so important and so intrinsic to human development that we cannot expose them to the vagaries and manipulations and inequities of the free market.

1. J. Michael Watt et al., "The Comparative Economic Performance of Investor-Owned Chain and Not-for-Profit Hospitals," *New England Journal of Medicine* 314:2, Jan. 9, 1986, pp. 89–96; Stephen Remm et al., "The Effects of Ownership and System Affiliation on the Economic Performance of Hospitals," *Inquiry* 22, Fall 1985, pp. 219–236; Arnold S. Relman, "Investor-Owned Hospitals and Health Care Costs," *New England Journal of Medicine* 309:54, Aug. 11, 1983, pp. 370–372; Daniel Ermann and John Gabel, "Multi Hospital Systems: Issues and Empirical Findings," *Health Affairs,* Spring 1984, pp. 50–64; Robert Pattison and Hallie Katz, "Investor-Owned and Not-For-Profit Hospitals: A Comparison Based on California Data," *New England Journal of Medicine* 309:53, Aug. 11, 1983, p. 347; B. Gordon, "For Profit Hospital Care: Who Profits, Who Cares?" National Council of Senior Citizens, 1986.
2. As the text indicates, values are discerned through an analysis of objective reality, not from feelings or emotions that are rationally indefensible. See Alisdar MacIntyre, *After Virtue,* University of Notre Dame Press, Notre Dame, IN, 1981.
3. Thomas Peters and Robert Waterman, *In Search of Excellence,* Warner Books, New York, 1983, p. 279.
4. President's Commission for the Study of Ethical Problems in Medicine and Biomedical and Behavioral Research, *Securing Access to Health Care,* 1983, especially Vols. II and III.
5. Peters and Waterman, p. 279.

6. Henrik Blum, *Planning for Health: Development and Application of Social Change,* Behavioral Publishers, New York, 1974, p. 93.
7. Blum, p. 96
8. Robert Merton, "Some Thoughts on Professions in American Society," unpublished paper presented at Brown University, 1960.
9. Kenneth Underwood, *The Church, the University and Social Policy,* Vol. 1, Wesleyan University Press, Middleton, CT, 1972, p. 422.
10. Edmund Pellegrino and David Thomasma, *A Philosophical Basis of Medical Practice,* Oxford University Press, New York, 1981, p. 23.
11. Charles Davidson, "Are We Physicians Helpless?" *New England Journal of Medicine* 310, Apr. 26, 1984, p. 1118.
12. For a detailed study in accord with this essay, see Gordon. For opinions contrary to this evaluation, see Richard Rosett, "Doing Well by Doing Good: Investor-Owned Hospitals," *Frontiers of Health Service Management,* 1, September 1984, pp. 1–9; Frank Sloan and Robert Vraciu, "Investor-Owned and Not-For-Profit Hospitals: Addressing Some Issues," *Health Affairs,* 2:1, 1983, pp. 25–37.
13. Eli Ginzberg, "The Grand Illusion of Competition in Health Care," and Council on Medical Services, American Medical Association, "Effects of Competition in Medicine," *Journal of American Medical Association,* 249:14, Apr. 18, 1983.
14. President's Commission, p. 20.
15. Eli Ginzberg, "The Monetarization of Medical Care," *New England Journal of Medicine* 310, May 3, 1984, p. 1163.
16. Unfortunately, some not-for-profit institutions are indistinguishable from investor-owned. See "Transfers to a Public Hospital," *New England Journal of Medicine* 314:9, Feb. 27, 1986, pp. 552–557.
17. President's Commission, pp. 22–23.
18. Paul Starr, *The Social Transformation of American Medicine,* Basic Books, New York, 1982, p. 448.
19. Michael Bromberg, quoted in "Conference on For-Profits," *AHA Washington Memo,* no. 494, March 16, 1984, p. 6.

20. See notes 1, 12, and 13.
21. Although the issue is not debated here, a significant difference exists between the interest on bonds paid by a not-for-profit corporation and the dividends paid to investors. See Kevin O'Rourke, "Investor-Owned Catholic Teaching Hospitals," *New England Journal of Medicine* 313:20, Nov. 14, 1985, p. 1297.
22. Starr, p. 448.
23. Arnold Relman, "The Commercialization of Medicine," unpublished paper presented to the Hospital Superintendents of New England, September 1983.
24. See note 16.
25. Starr, p. 446.

General Principles of Medical Ethics

Part II

Genetic Screening: Do People Really Want to Know Their Future?   **10**

Genetic screening for some diseases has been possible for several years. Genetic screening can be done for individuals or couples who anticipate having a child and wish to know their genetic makeup and what genetic diseases might affect their offspring.

Genetic screening is done prenatally to determine medical difficulties that children suffer in utero. In a few cases, treatments can help the fetus. In almost all cases, psychological and social support structures can be established for parents to prepare for the birth of a child with genetic anomalies.

In addition, newborn testing for some genetic diseases, such as phenylketonuria (PKU), is done for most children born in the United States. PKU is a metabolic disease that, when identified at the time of birth, can be treated through dietary restrictions so a child suffers no adverse affects. PKU testing is one example of genetic screening that provides information that benefits a child's health.

Newborn, prenatal, and adult screening provides people with information that is helpful in personal decisions. This raises many legal and ethical concerns, from abortion for the child screened prenatally and found to have a genetic disorder, to confidentiality of test results, to sharing of test results with third parties such as family members.

These issues are heightened by the development of more complex chromosomal tests for diseases such as Huntington's disease or cystic fibrosis.

The questions raised with the new, complex chromosomal tests are similar to those that already exist in a variety of other genetic screening programs. What testing should be done? When should testing be done? Who has a right to the information of the tests? How is the information used? Can people be forced into testing programs? What are the consequences of discovering the possibility or certainty of genetic disease, such as Huntington's disease, especially for adults later in life?

The impact of genetic discoveries, treatment for genetic disease, screening programs, and other related concerns require all healthcare facilities to address the issue of genetics. These issues can be discussed at the time of a proposal for genetic screening or when other genetic concerns arise in the institution.

In February 1983 the President's Commission for the Study of Ethical Problems in Medicine and Biomedical and Behavioral Research published a study entitled *Screening and Counseling for Genetic Conditions: The Ethical, Social, and Legal Implications of Genetic Screening, Counseling, and Education Programs.*[1] The ethical principles outlined by the commission guide not only existing prenatal newborn testing or adult screening, but also give direction to future genetic concerns. The main ethical principles are "autonomy, beneficence (including the prevention of harm), justice (including equity and fairness), and privacy (including confidentiality)."

Confidentiality

The first ethical issue is confidentiality. The President's Commission states "because of the potential for misuse as well as unintended social or economic injury, information from genetic testing should be given to people such as insurers or employers only with the explicit consent of the person screened."[2] Confidentiality is designed to enhance the relationship between the healthcare provider and the patient. Also, confidentiality protects information exchanged in the physician-patient relationship from those outside that relationship.

Screening of any type raises difficult issues because the information obtained through screening can be used to discriminate unjustly against individuals in the job market, housing, and health and life insurance. Tension arises in the insurance area because health and life insurance premiums are meant to establish an equitable distribution of costs for healthcare across a wide range of the population. When individuals at risk for genetic disease and higher costs are not accounted for properly, other individuals may be required to pay a greater premium. Should individuals at risk for serious illness have higher premiums to offset higher costs at a later time? The difficulty is that not all individuals at risk for specific diseases necessarily contract the disease. Thus, those at risk for heart disease or cancer, penalized by higher premiums because of family history, may never collect on those premiums because they do not develop the disease.

The more complex chromosomal test available for Huntington's disease provides definitive information about whether or not one will contract the disease. Should the person identified be required to pay higher insurance premiums, or should the person be denied health insurance because of the certainty of illness? Does information that definitively identifies one as a person who will suffer from an illness in the future require that the individual pay substantially higher insurance premiums? Or should these patients be considered as part of a larger population, thus spreading financial risks more equitably? These ethical issues are not easily answered.

Housing, employment, and other basic values are threatened by recorded data if confidentiality is not maintained. What can be developed, given contemporary computer data systems, to ensure that inappropriate persons do not gain access to confidential information?

Confidentiality becomes more difficult, however, when individuals who are aware of their at-risk problems through genetic screening refuse to share the information with other family members who may also be at risk. The chromosomal tests for Huntington's disease are an example. If one's parent contracts Huntington's disease, there is a 50 percent chance that each child will also develop the disease. Screening a child, who is the offspring of an adult whose parent has Huntington's disease can give positive information about both the child and the child's parent. If the at-risk parent has refused information how does one handle the information, from the genetics test done on the child? Should this information be shared? If a prenatal test is positive, the at-risk parent also is positive for that condition. Should the information be kept secret? If not, how does one justify giving information in some circumstances but not in others? Does the physician or genetic counselor have a responsibility to share information? Institutions that offer sophisticated genetic screening as a service for their patients must address these issues before the start of a program. The complications, however, should not preclude the institution's involvement in beneficial healthcare technologies.

It is necessary to maintain confidentiality while outlining those instances where a professional or an institution may breach confidentiality to protect others. The President's Commission suggests that confidentiality be breached only if reasonable efforts to elicit voluntary consent to the disclosure of information have been tried and refused by the affected individual. Also, if the information is withheld there must be a high probability that the harm to another person can be avoided and beneficial medical treatment provided. Even though this suggestion is adopted in some circles, delineating the lines of harm and identifying what benefits will accrue to another individual when confidentiality is broken are difficult to determine.

Autonomy

A second ethical principle identified by the President's Commission is autonomy. Are people free to enter or not to enter genetic counseling and screening programs? Or should there be societally based programs over which an individual has no choice? Presently, both situations exist.

In the case of PKU, mandatory screening is required for every newborn child, because it can alleviate all the detrimental effects that PKU will have for a child. The treatment is not expensive, is easily administered, and does not require sophisticated equipment. Ethically, this mandatory testing is acceptable because of the availability of the test and the ability to provide beneficial treatment.

This is not the case for Huntington's disease. People who test positive under the new protocols for the Huntington's disease marker do not have any option about contracting the disease. If they test positive, they will be affected later in life.

There is no cure. Can society or the medical community force this information on individuals? Is it acceptable not to know and to wait until the disease strikes? Ethically, certainty about the disease with no possible beneficial treatment, other than psychological and social support, makes testing a voluntary matter.

An informed choice by an individual whether or not to undergo a particular genetic test should be respected, except in those programs where beneficial treatment is available. The norm for genetic screening and counseling is *voluntary*. Individuals should not be tested to maximize social values or to save dollars by not allocating resources to those who are ill or will become ill with a disease that cannot be cured. To create structures of prejudice and injustice for those at risk for genetic diseases is unethical. The President's Commission states: "In sum, the fundamental value of genetic screening and counseling is their ability to enhance the opportunities for individuals to obtain information about their personal health and childbearing risks and to make autonomous and noncoerced choices based on that information."[3]

Beneficence

Beneficence, another ethical principle, means that a health-care endeavor provides benefits rather than harm for a patient. Mandatory or elective genetic screening for individuals raises questions about the existing physiological, psychological, and social benefits. Are there benefits obtained for the patient through the provision of information? This is the dividing line between mandatory testing programs, such as for PKU, and optional testing programs, such as for Huntington's disease.

When little can be done for an individual, as with Huntington's disease, the obligation that individuals at risk be tested, on a mandatory basis, seems unjust. More harm than benefit can result from the test. Some individuals will want to know about the future of their health, which may have an impact on decisions about reproduction, jobs, insurance, or marriage. Others in the same situation may wish to go on with life assuming they will be healthy and experience normal adulthood;

they may want to deal with a disease issue only when initial symptoms develop. Voluntary programs provide for both types of individuals.

The ethical commitments of society attempt to balance the well-being of the community with the well-being and autonomy of the individual. A commitment to the principle of beneficience in genetic screening and counseling requires flexibility to allow individuals to make choices according to their personal needs and idiosyncratic choices. Social support should be given to individuals in both circumstances.

Justice

Justice, another issue, is a difficult concept to define. Within the arena of genetic screening and counseling, justice means that there will be an equitable distribution of the risks and benefits involved in a screening program.

Violations of justice and equity principles are evident in the different ways testing was done concerning sickle-cell anemia for blacks and Tay-Sachs disease for Ashkenazim Jews. The social support structures developed for the Ashkenazim Jews through synagogues. Community organizations provided comfort, support, and medical care necessary for those who received information about Tay-Sachs disease and the risks to their offspring. In the black community, sickle-cell anemia testing did not pay attention to similar supportive details. As a result, people received important information about reproductive concerns without the social, economic, and medical support available in Tay-Sachs testing.

The lesson of the testing programs should alert healthcare institutions of the need to develop protocols that include care for individuals beyond the testing and information exchanged by physicians, counselors, and other appropriate personnel. Continued supportive care will be needed as people understand the information and make choices. Equity is a concern about the information given and access to services available for the person at a later time. Genetic information that is given with an assumption of moral failure or blame, especially for couples who decide to have children, is unacceptable. As the President's Commission states in its conclusions, equity is best served when screening programs for any population reflect the balance of benefits and harms. These in turn also should reflect the incidence of the disease within the population and the ability to provide care for that population later. Information about a disease for which no healthcare services are available is inequitable.[4]

Conclusion

Knowing one's genetic history is an important part of other decisions that one makes in life regarding jobs, family, and children. The development of genetic screening and counseling to date, however, is not best served by requiring that every person have a complete set of facts about their own genetic history or by requiring that those individuals who may be at risk receive such information. The future of the delivery of preventive healthcare services in all healthcare institutions will increasingly move toward the provision of genetic information. As healthcare institutions confront these issues, they must have an established forum, such as ethics committees, to discuss these and a variety of other issues. All genetics programs should reflect the mission of the institution; the dignity, value, and worth of human life; and the provision of services that benefit individuals.

1. President's Commission for the Study of Ethical Problems in Medicine and Biomedical and Behavioral Research, *Screening and Counseling for Genetic Conditions: The Ethical, Social, and Legal Implications of Genetic Screening, Counseling, and Education Programs*, Government Printing Office, Washington, DC, 1983.

2. President's Commission, p. 42.
3. President's Commission, p. 55.
4. President's Commission, pp. 75–86.

Making Healthcare Decisions 11
for Others

On Sept. 11, 1986, the State Supreme Court of Massachusetts ruled that the feeding tube that kept Paul Brophy "alive" for three and a half years could be removed and that his wishes not to live in a persistent vegetative state should be respected.

The court's decision deals with many ethical issues. In part, the decision addresses the problems raised by a previously competent patient who has made known his or her wishes to accept or reject certain medical treatments. Also, the ruling tries to protect the values of an individual hospital by not requiring the hospital to follow procedures that it finds ethically reprehensible. The decision also allows the hospital to transfer the patient to another institution where both the patient's values and the institution's moral commitment will be respected.

Cases such as Paul Brophy's can involve ethics committees on a consultative basis. The ethics committee may not replace the courts or the development of law but they can help people to think through the various ethical dimensions of these decisions.

The Values of Decision Making

Decision making for incompetent patients employs the principle of proxy consent. The principle requires that the decision maker decide for the incompetent person as that person would have decided for himself or herself. The temptation for many decision makers, however, is to make decisions for the incompetent patient as they think they should be made, or in accordance with their own emotional needs, wishes, or feelings.

Paul Brophy was an incompetent patient who left clear evidence of what it was that he wanted. In previous conversations with his family and others, he clearly indicated that he did not wish to have life-sustaining procedures maintained if he were deprived of mental function and it seemed he would not recover. Such statements help clarify a formerly competent patient's wishes. The assumption of the proxy consent principle is that the values that would be expressed in the dialogue between the healthcare provider and the competent patient still will be respected. If all incompetent patients were individuals who had formerly been competent and who had clearly expressed the values that they wished to see realized in their healthcare decisions, these issues would be less complicated.

Advance directives in the form of living wills, generally very limited in scope, are one attempt to communicate personal values so that when difficult decisions are made at the end of life, some indication of patient preference is available. The difficulty with living wills is that they are usually restricted to the terminally ill, incompetent, or imminently dying person. However, many incompetent patients who need decisions made for them do not fall into this category. Although living wills are ethically sound documents for end-of-life decisions for a limited group of patients, they are not very helpful for other individuals.

Frequently, an incompetent patient has not made his or her wishes known previous to the time of incompetency, or the person has never been competent to make decisions. Thus, it is impossible to identify what decisions a person would make at the time in question. Ethics committees may then be consulted on the appropriate stages one uses to make a decision for an incompetent patient.

The Role of Ethics Committees

When institutional ethics committees (IECs) are asked to participate in discussions that involve decisions for an incompetent patient, the committee's proper focus is on understanding the values of the patient and the elements of good medical decision making. The IEC should address certain value statements. First: What did the individual want? What was valued in life? What actions or activities are clear expressions of the patient's values? These questions require that the individual was clear about the importance of medical care, the value of life, religious preferences, and other kinds of values.

The second question is: What decision would this person have made if capable of making the decision now? Although the principle seems clear, implementing it is difficult. Difficulties arise because no particular medical scenario is entirely imagined by an individual before a medical crisis occurs. It is impossible for an individual to articulate clearly what he or she would want in every situation. Frequently, ambiguity or indecision is easily identified. It is a mistake to walk into the ethical discussion about decision making for an incompetent patient with a presumed sense that clarity and preciseness are established.

The third question involves the ambiguity of medicine itself. IECs have to remember that medicine is not an exact science and cannot "promise" certain results. Many medical decisions have to be made in the midst of ambiguity about the medical condition of the individual, the prognosis, and the promise of a therapeutic intervention. Working through this ambiguity is one of the most important tasks IECs can perform. In fact, the ability to raise and discuss the various facets of the issue is the strength of the ethics committee discussion.

It is wrong for the IEC to become the medical decision maker. The membership of the committee represents excellence in a variety of disciplines. It is difficult, however, for this interdisciplinary body to have the expertise necessary to make an appropriate decision for the patient. The heart of medicine is the relationship between the provider and the patient, which is not embodied in the IEC.

The ethics committee, however, may provide a forum for consultation. Consultation is not a request for a medical decision. Physicians, healthcare providers, and institutions should not push IECs into that position. Rather, consultation is the recognition that, in decision making for incompetent patients, the expertise of a variety of disciplines can be helpful.

The membership of the IEC must be clear about the medical realities and ambiguities of a particular case. In addition, members must be clear about the values of the individual and the family involved. The values of the patient may not be the same as those of the family members, and the values of the patient may not be the same as many, or all, of the IEC members. Consequently, the ethics committee must be open to differences in value structures, especially in a pluralistic society. If the committee is not able to do this, it will not be a helpful structure.

Conclusion

The case of Paul Brophy raises issues in nutrition and hydration, but it also serves as an example of the values involved in decision making for incompetent patients not covered by living wills. The law cannot develop statutory laws to cover all cases of medical decision making for incompetent patients. Thus, institutions must develop a method by which the values involved in these decisions can be discussed, explored, and understood.

IECs can provide a forum for discussion that identifies appropriate values, explores possible solutions, educates possible solutions, educates professional care givers, and alleviates unnecessary future problems. IECs will not keep cases out of the courts but can help minimize the times that legal recourse is necessary.

The Capacity for Healthcare   12
Decision Making

Competency is one factor considered when determining an individual's ability to participate in a decision-making process. Competency is required to make decisions about many matters, including healthcare. The more serious the impact of the decision on life, the more competent one expects the decision maker to be. The capacity for patients to share in this decision-making process in healthcare is a concern for many professionals.

There are many ways in which people judge whether or not a person is competent to make a healthcare decision. Identifying the criteria an individual uses to determine the competency of an individual patient is central. The temptation is to identify one specific criterion for all health-related decision-making settings, as opposed to structuring sliding-scale criteria that depend on the person, the medical condition, and the type of decision required.

Criteria of Choice

One way people determine whether or not an individual is competent is based on the choice the individual makes. The rationale is that competent people make wise choices; an unwise choice indicates incompetency. Wise choices exhibit a preference for the value of life, an appreciation of health, or an acceptance of medical treatments. When people make choices that are not in accord with these predetermined values, their competency is questioned.

People who choose to die rather than to live, people who choose to withhold or withdraw certain medical treatments rather than continue them, and people who choose against some psychiatric or medical treatments are judged incompetent based on their choice. Once an individual is declared incompetent, then a "rational choice" is made by a guardian.

Some values, such as the value of life, are recognized as universally important. However, because one chooses not to pursue life at all costs does not mean that a person is incompetent. Likewise, because one agrees to a specific choice does not mean a person is competent. A choice in and of itself cannot bear the weight of competency determinations.

Category Criteria

Some people make competency decisions based on "categories" of patients. As a result, all patients who suffer from a life-threatening illness are incompetent to make decisions. People who are old or who are placed in an institutionalized setting, such as a long term care facility, are incompetent to make choices. Those who have a history of psychiatric treatment are not competent.

Undoubtedly, one can declare some "categories" of patients as incompetent. The categories include neonates, children before the age of reason, and individuals who are in a persistent vegetative state. The mistake is to believe that competency or incompetency is a result of being in one of these categories. The reason these people are incompetent is because they are not capable of entering into a consensual discussion to make decisions.

Consistency of Values

Other people require a consistency-of-value choice across time for a person to be competent. People look to the past and ask questions about the values expressed by the patient through time. The consistency of statements and the certainty one has about the continued value preferences of a patient indicate the patient's competency in the present setting.

The difficulty with this criterion is that it does not allow individuals the freedom to change their preferences with their experience of illness or medical treatment. Not infrequently, individuals who have stated that they would always want to receive aggressive treatment find that a particular disease is so debilitating or a particular therapy so burdensome that, although this was a consistent choice in the past, it is no longer their present desire. A shift in personal values occurs.

Likewise, other individuals reflect on a series of therapeutic procedures provided to family members and consistently state that they would not want such therapies. When illness strikes, however, or when people are confronted with a life-and-death situation, they embrace life more radically and change their mind about their previous refusal of medical treatment.

To state that individuals must maintain one choice, and that competency is measured on that basis, is to deny the reality of experience and persons' ability to change in response to it. Competency should not require this strait-jacket approach.

A Sliding Scale

The difficulty with these criteria is the identification of one criterion for all circumstances. The more difficult task is to identify and use sliding-scale criteria for competency. Drane wrote about a set of standards he labeled Standard 1, Standard 2, and Standard 3 that should be used when questioning a person's competence.[1]

In Drane's opinion, the less severe the consequences of the choices made by the patient, the less demanding should be the criteria for competency. Individuals who have low-risk and low-benefit consequences from a particular therapy, which they choose or refuse, should not have stringent requirements of competency placed on them. Preferences should be respected. On the other end of the scale, when a choice to omit or to proceed with a particular therapy has a great impact on life or means the difference between life and death, severe criteria of understanding and comprehension should be required of persons because of the nature and severity of the consequences of their choices.

What Drane suggests is the development of an elastic concept of competency. Factors such as "benefit," "risk," "knowledge," "understanding," and "deep appreciation" are the measuring stick of competency. The less severe the consequences to the person, the less comprehensive an understanding is required. The more severe the consequences, the fuller the comprehension required.

Prudential judgments by the healthcare professional are required when making competency decisions. The physician must balance the patient's ability to understand, the realistic consequences of the choices made, and the present situation.

In summary, the focus for competency is (1) what is the patient asked to choose, (2) what participatory abilities does he or she have when making this choice, and (3) what are the nature and severity of the consequences of the choices. Competent individuals can make choices at one level but can be denied the ability to make choices at another, depending on the circumstances.

Other Considerations about Competency

The decision-making capacity of a patient is always presumed. When individuals make statements, choices, or exhibit behavior that does not seem to be consistent with a competent choice, the statements indicate the need for a competency investigation and not that a person is automatically incompetent. Careful evaluations by appropriate healthcare personnel are then conducted to determine whether or not the individual is able to understand and comprehend the information provided and the consequences of the decisions made in the particular situation. Competency investigations measure the ability of patients to understand what is wrong with them, weigh various alternatives, and appreciate the consequences of their choices in a given setting.

Sliding-scale criteria are important because a patient's cognitive abilities may be sharp on one day and dull on another, making the day of discussion as important an element in the decision-making process as the patient's cognitive capacities. A sole criterion for competency denies the values that informed consent seeks to realize.

Conclusion

Competency is one of the fundamental requirements of informed consent. The competency of individuals to make healthcare decisions has to be carefully measured. The ultimate goal of competency decisions is to protect the value of patient participation in healthcare decisions.

---

1. James Drane, "The Many Faces of Competency," *Hastings Center Report*, April 1985, pp. 17-26.

On Playing God   13

Consider the situation where guests appearing on a radio or TV talk show devoted to questions of medical ethics or health-care professionals discuss a difficult patient-care decision in a clinical setting. If the proposed ethical solution suggests that a person be allowed to die, someone will object to the solution and say, "You are playing God." This phrase is usually uttered with the implied meaning: "Life and death decisions in medical care must be left to God. Human beings have no right to interfere with God's work." Is this a reasonable attitude? Is there any sense in which human beings can and should "play God?" Or should human beings be more cautious, withdrawing from decision making when it becomes obvious that death might unavoidably ensue if another good is chosen? Understanding the concept "on playing God" will help us understand better the mission, nobility, and limits of medicine.

Principle

The term *God* implies an all-powerful, wise, and good being whom human beings worship as creator and ruler of the universe (*Webster's Dictionary*). God is the provident director of events and happenings in the universe. Those who do not believe in a personal God might substitute for God the term *Nature*, meaning "a creative and controlling force in the universe" (*Webster's Dictionary*).

Is there any sense in which human beings ought "to play God" or "assume the role of nature?" The glory and challenge of being human is that we are called on "to play God": we are challenged to assist nature by being creative and by controlling our own lives and the happenings of the environment. If we are to fulfill our humanity, we must take an active role in shaping our own destiny, help others fulfill their destiny, and maintain the ecology of the universe. We are created in the image and likeness of God. We have powers from God (Nature), our intellect and our will, that enable us to take an active and determining role in the decisions affecting our lives and our destinies. We can respect and develop our person and capacities, whether mental or physical, or allow them to deteriorate and atrophy. We can build great societies or allow ourselves to destroy one another through bitterness, envy, and violence. We can respect our environment and preserve it for generations to come, or we can ravage it rapaciously and leave a wasteland for our progeny.

Medical research is an illustrious example of our ability and need "to play God." Medical research seeks to improve human life by eliminating disease and improving our quality of life. Would it be fitting for the medical community to remain passive in face of the AIDS epidemic and say, "This is God's way of punishing people and we must not interfere." Of course not. Rather, the medical research community, at the behest of all caring people, plays God and tries to eliminate AIDS, thus controlling the future and eventually eliminating one more source of human suffering.

In medical matters, most people realize the need to be responsible for personal health. Realizing that they cannot expect God to send medical care unless they do something about seeking out this help, most people will seek medical help if they are ill. Few people realize, however, that we have the power and responsibility to be creative and controlling in regard to other facets of medical care. For example, by working together, we can do something to provide more adequate healthcare for all members of our society. Moreover, through mutual cooperation, we can improve our environment and the quality of life in our cities.

Although we have the power to play God, or influence Nature, regarding our personal, social, and ecological responsibilities, we do not have unlimited power. God has unlimited power, but to be human is to be limited. Unfortunately, admitting limitations and shortcomings seems to be difficult for human beings. If we choose one goal, it usually means we must relinquish another. By choosing to avoid physical or mental suffering, one with a fatal pathology may also reject lifeprolonging therapy and thus hasten death. We cannot "have it all." "Playing God" in the sense of not admitting limitations leads ultimately to personal unhappiness and social disaster. Thus, we are called on to play God insofar as being creative and planning for the future is concerned. To realize this power responsibly, however, we must recognize our limitations.

Discussion

In medical care, the tendency to ignore subconsciously the limitations of knowledge and technique is prevalent.[1] Some physicians, for example, act as though the death of a patient is a personal defeat. Thus, physicians themselves testify that those who have incurable and terminal disease often are not given the same attention as those who may recover from their illness. Given the limitations of human beings, helping people die well is just as much a part of medical care as healing. Knowing when to cure and when to "simply care" is the epitome of the science and art of medicine.

Admitting limitations for research programs is also difficult. Do those who set policy for research programs stop to say, "We can't do everything; what are the most beneficial things we can do with our limited resources"? Rather, it seems that political economic pressures determine the research agenda. In the United States, medical care and research programs emphasize experimental procedures for the few, such as transplants and artificial organs, whereas more basic programs for the many, such as neonatal care, often are neglected. Medical progress requires that some attention be given to experimental procedures, but are policies on research and practice formulated with a view to social as well as personal medical needs? A neutral observer evaluating U.S. research programs' medical practice might state, "These programs are based on the assumptions that medical care can enable people to live forever and that there are unlimited financial resources."

Besides healthcare professionals, the general public also often presumes that no limitations exist to healthcare funding. Many consider it an egregious violation of human rights if a representative of a healthcare facility, especially a Catholic facility, is forced to say, "I am sorry, we don't have the funds to accept you as a patient." True, healthcare institutions, especially Catholic ones, by reason of the profession to which they are dedicated, should do as much charity care as possible. Institutions as well as individual persons have limits, however, and it is not a violation of others' rights if facilities acknowledge publicly these limits.

Conclusion

Playing God in a worthwhile sense means that we realize we are responsible for the destiny of ourselves, others, and the environment. But it also means that, in fulfilling our responsibilities, we must admit our limitatons. Admitting limitations is simply another way of saying that we must pose the relevant ethical questions:
- If we can't do everything, what goods or values are more important than others?
- Which research and therapy programs should receive priority? What must we give up in order to provide more equitable access to healthcare?

---

1. Eugene D. Robin, *Matters of Life and Death*, Freeman Co., New York, 1984, p. 179.

Physicians: Healers or Officers 14
of the Court?

The patient arrives in the emergency room, dazed, badly injured, and accompanied by a policeman. The policeman insists that the attending physician draw blood from the accident victim to evaluate whether she was driving while intoxicated. The patient resists having blood drawn. Should the emergency room personnel immobilize the patient and draw the blood anyway?

In addition to the more dramatic occurrences when physicians are requested or required to test accident victims for the presence of debilitating substances in their blood, such as alcohol or cocaine, there are also less urgent programs for drug testing. In these programs the entire work force of a company might be subjected to testing because of a mandate issued by an employer; employees are selected at random for testing. Should physicians take part in programs that call for random drug testing? What role should the physician play in regard to detecting people who break the law or who may endanger their own lives and the lives of others? What responsibility do physicians have to act as agents of the court?

Principles

Clearly, there are people who endanger themselves and others by operating automobiles and other machines in an impaired condition. In addition, there are people who break the law by using prohibited substances. Surveys indicate that more than half of the automobile accidents involve drivers who are under the influence of alcohol. Industrial accidents also involve a significant percentage of people who are impaired by alcohol or other psychoactive substances. Society has a right and a responsibility to protect human lives and eliminate the incidence of accidents that involve people who are debilitated because of the abusing of mind-altering substances. Physicians, as responsible members of society, should cooperate in an effort to preserve life and limit injuries.

To conduct drug testing in an ethical manner, however, and to protect the rights of physicians and the rights of individuals, some clear distinctions are needed. Although society has rights to protect life and promote safety, society does not have absolute rights. Citizens have rights as well. Even though employers have a right to require competent and industrious employees, the rights of employers are not absolute. Employees have rights as well.

The fundamental rights of an individual, whether the individual is considered as a citizen, an employee, or even a patient, stems from the individual's human worth and dignity. The fundamental right to treatment as a person of worth and integrity is not bestowed by society, employers, or physicians. Rather, it springs from the person's existence as a human being. When considering how to protect life and promote safety, therefore, the programs in question must consider the worth of the individual person. The argument is often put forward that people who do not break the law have nothing to fear from drug testing. Thus drug testing should be allowed and should be mandatory. This argument overlooks, however, that proving one's innocence when one is not guilty of substance abuse is a demeaning experience. In the United States we have a legal principle, "A person is innocent until proven guilty." The roots of this dictum go beyond law to the very heart of human worth. Demanding that one prove innocence when there is no cause to suspect guilt devastates self-esteem, a touchstone of human worth and integrity. In sum, the individual does not surrender his or her fundamental right to be respected as a person of worth simply because one becomes a citizen of a particular society, is employed by a company or business, or becomes a patient in need of medical care.

In regard to fostering human worth, physicians have a special responsibility. The profession of the healing arts must involve a relationship founded on trust. Thus, the patient must be convinced that the physician or other healthcare professional is interested in him or her, and that the fundamental and primary cause of this interest is the physician's desire to protect and heal the patient. If the patient considers the physician primarily as an agent of the court or someone interested primarily in making money, then the potential for a relationship built on trust is weakened, if not destroyed.

Discussion

When acting as healers in the emergency room or any other place, physicians must balance the rights of the patient, the rights of society, and their own rights. If a person is an accident victim and suspected of driving while intoxicated, the primary goal of the physician must be to heal the injured person. If the law officer requests some procedure be performed that would provide evidence in a trial, then the physician in question must observe the norms of informed consent. If the patient is unconscious, then it seems no procedures should be performed that would incriminate the patient. If a person is unconscious, only those procedures may be performed to which the patient would consent were he or she conscious. May we presume that unconscious accident victims would want their blood drawn to be tested by a police laboratory?

The point is not that an accident victim suspected of driving while intoxicated should never be tested by competent authority. Rather, the point is that such testing should not be performed by physicians unless there is informed consent or the basis for presumed consent. If some semblance of informed consent is not present when gathering evidence is proposed by an officer of the law, then the healthcare professionals become agents of the court, pure and simple, and weaken the acceptance of medicine as a healing profession. Gathering legal evidence does not necessarily require the cooperation of physicians. The courts have many ways of assessing the competence of a driver and of gathering evidence, even evidence requiring hematological studies.

Concerning other forms of testing, the physician must also be careful to respect the rights of individuals. Random drug screening is ethically acceptable only if the people being tested are responsible for the public good in a direct manner, for example, if they are responsible for the lives and safety of many people. Thus, airline pilots and bus drivers might be groups who would be candidates for random screening, although a record of safety over a length of time might exempt people from such programs. Random screening programs that are justified only because drugs are illegal, however, do not seem to be ethically acceptable, since they involve a method of enforcing the law that is personally demeaning. Physicians should not take part in such programs lest they mitigate the meaning of their own profession.

Sometimes a person who has not been injured, but who has been involved in an industrial accident, is presented for testing accompanied by an employer or a shop steward. Such testing may be in accord with a union or employment contract. Even in these cases, informed consent should be required. Again, the rights of the employee, the union, and the employer to have the testing performed are not under question. Rather, the question is, how should such testing be performed ethically by a physician?

Conclusion

Some of the conclusions of this essay are not in accord with accepted medical practice. If physicians are not concerned about values evidenced in the practice of medicine, however, no one else will be. Thus, the previous considerations foster two important values:

1. The value of the individual as a person possessing fundamental rights not granted by society, employer, or physician

2. The value of medicine as a healing profession based on a relationship of trust

The AMA Statement on Tube   15
Feeding: An Ethical Analysis

On March 15, 1986, the Council on Ethical and Judicial Affairs of the American Medical Association (AMA) issued a statement declaring that life-prolonging medical treatment and artifically or technologically supplied respiration, nutrition, and hydration may be withheld from a patient in an irreversible coma "even if death is not imminent."[1] The statement seems to be ethically acceptable, but it has been seriously questioned by some and rejected by others.

For example, the rationale for the AMA statement was not being followed by the lower courts in the recent *Brophy* case in Massachusetts, in which Judge H. David Kopelman was petitioned to allow removal of the tube feeding from a patient diagnosed as irreversibly comatose. Wisely seeking to base his legal decision on ethical consensus, Judge Kopelman interviewed several physicians and ethicists. Finding no consensus, he stated that Paul Brophy, then in an irreversible coma, would have desired to have all life-support systems removed. But he determined that: "It is ethically inappropriate to cause the preventable death of Brophy by the deliberate denial of food and water that can be provided to him in a noninvasive, nonintrusive manner that causes no pain and suffering, irrespective of the substituted judgment of the patient."[2] Thus, Judge Kopelman focused on the amount of suffering involved, not the condition of the patient, to justify the continuation of tube feeding.

In New Jersey, the *Jobes* case attracts our attention because the lawyers arguing for the nursing home where Nancy Jobes was maintained on artificial hydration and nutrition rejected the reasoning of the AMA statement, declaring that life support should not be withdrawn because Mrs. Jobes was "not terminally ill." Although the Superior Court of Morris County, NJ, decided on March 16, 1986, to allow nutrition and hydration to be withdrawn from Mrs. Jobes, the argument of the lawyers representing the nursing home is significant because many pro-life advocates agree with it.

In both the *Brophy* and *Jobes* cases, the Supreme Courts of the states of Massachusetts and New Jersey allowed artificial hydration and nutrition to be withdrawn from the comatose persons. While these decisions do not answer all the ethical issues involved, they demonstrate a developing consensus toward the issue of when to remove life support from people in a persistent vegetative state.

Finally, while admitting "that means for providing nourishment may become too ineffective or burdensome to be obligatory," a recent statement of the U.S. Bishops' Committee for Pro-Life Activities states a strong presumption in favor of their use.[3]

The purpose of this essay is to resolve some of the controversy that surrounds the withholding of artificial nutrition and hydration in general, and the AMA statement in particular. In the course of the article, we consider some distinctions that may help develop ethical consensus and on which legal decisions may be based.

Imminent Death

Among the confusing factors in determining ethical healthcare for seriously ill patients are the phrases "imminent death" and "terminal condition." These phrases are often invoked as though they determine a patient's medical care. For example, in the Karen Ann Quinlan and Paul Brophy cases, imminence of death was considered an important issue. In general, the terms imminent death and terminal condition imply that a physician can predict that a patient will die of a fatal pathology within a few days or weeks no matter what life-prolonging methods are employed. Using these terms as significant factors in making ethical and legal decisions begs the question. The important issue is not how long the patient might live with life-support systems, but whether the life-support systems should be applied to seriously ill patients in the first place.

Aside from murder and suicide, death occurs from a pathology internal to the physiological system that so unbalances homeostasis that the patient cannot survive. Life-prolonging therapy such as surgery for cancer, aims at removing a potentially fatal pathology by circumventing or delaying the effect of the fatal pathology. Thus, a person on kidney dialysis has a fatal pathology, but the effects of the pathology are circumvented by dialysis. By definition, a patient in an irreversible coma cannot eat and swallow and thus will die of that pathology in a short time unless life-prolonging devices are used to circumvent the pathology. Withholding artificial hydration and nutrition from a patient in an irreversible coma does not induce a new fatal pathology; rather, it allows an already existing fatal pathology to take its natural course.

Basis for Ethical Obligation

How does one decide either to treat a fatal pathology or to let it take its natural course? One of the basic ethical assumptions on which medicine and efforts to nurse and feed people are based is that life should be prolonged because living enables us to pursue the purpose of life. Thus, we assume that an ethical obligation exists to prolong life. But does that obligation ever cease? Clearly, it would cease if prolonging life does not contribute to striving for the purpose of life. If efforts to prolong life are useless or result in a severe burden for the patient insofar as the pursuing the purpose of life is concerned, then the ethical obligation to prolong life is no longer present.

Useless Therapy

In order to pursue the purpose of life, one needs some degree of cognitive-affective function. Although the argument will not be developed here, the various definitions people offer for the purpose of life—happiness, fulfillment, love of God and neighbor, human relationships—imply some ability to function at the cognitive-affective, or spiritual, level. Thus, if efforts to restore cognitive-affective function in an adult can be judged useless, or if it can be judged that an infant will never develop cognitive-affective function, and if a fatal pathology is present, the adult or infant may be allowed to die. There is no need to seek to remove the fatal pathology or to circumvent its effects if the efforts would not enable the individual to achieve cognitive-affective function and strive for the purpose of life. This is the precise ethical justification for discontinuing artificial hydration and nutrition for people in an irreversible coma, not the fact "that benefits of treatment outweigh its burdens," as the AMA statement seems to indicate.

Physiological function, which can be prolonged long after cognitive-affective function ceases irreparably, is not a sufficient reason for prolonging life. Physiological function bereft of the potential for cognitive-affective function does not benefit the patient and does not contribute to pursuing the purpose of life. The primary role of physiological function is to support cognitive-affective function, but we know physiological activity can continue long after cognitive-affective function is irreparably lost.

Is the person who has physiological function but no hope of recovering cognitive-affective function still a human being? Yes, but there is no ethical obligation to strive to prolong the life of that human being. An ethical obligation does exist to keep the person comfortable; we have more to say about comfort care. However, the usual ethical obligation to prolong the life of another person when a fatal pathology is present ceases once it can be determined that the person will never recover, or initially develop, cognitive-affective function.

Notice that the pain, or lack of it, associated with the life-prolonging therapy is not in itself a significant ethical factor when considering whether the therapy is useful or useless in regard to restoring cognitive-affective function. For this reason, Judge Kopelman's decision is flawed, because life-prolonging therapy should be withdrawn as soon as it is obvious that it is useless in restoring cognitive-affective function. The degree of pain is not per se a consideration in the ethical decision concerning useless therapy; neither should it influence the legal decision concerning the same issue. The degree of pain may influence the decision concerning the burden that prolonging life may entail, but not concerning the usefulness or uselessness of life-prolonging therapy.

Grave Burden

Whether prolonging life will result in a grave burden insofar as striving for the purpose of life is concerned is more difficult to determine. Simply because the ethical decision is more difficult and complex, however, does not mean it is to be rejected or supplanted by a law that eliminates consideration of some meaningful circumstances. If the person with a fatal pathology is competent, then he or she should be allowed to make the decision, based on ethical norms, whether or not to prolong life. Thus, the seriously ill person is not "autonomous" in the absolute sense as some court decisions and ethicists would seem to indicate. The decision about prolonging life should take all personal, familial, and social circumstances into account because one has responsibility to self, family, and society in fulfilling the purpose of life.

For example, a father whose life is threatened because of cancer may decide that his purpose in life would be better fulfilled if he rejected chemotherapy, surgery, or hospitalization in order to devote his time to his family during his remaining days and to devote his savings toward the education of his children. Given the circumstances, the father is not "choosing death." Rather, realizing that he must die sometime, he determines that it is spiritually more beneficial for him to die in the immediate future, rather than to prolong his life for 2, 3, or even 10 years and as a result endanger other values, such as meaningful time with loved ones or the education of his children.

Once again, the severity or lack of pain is not the determining factor in making the decision whether or not to prolong life. What we seek to assess when making this ethical decision is the burden that would result if life is prolonged, not the burden that the therapy used to prolong life would involve. This distinction seems to be misunderstood by many ethicists and judges. Many ask, when faced with the decision of whether or not to prolong the life of another, "Will the therapy be painful?" The burden under discussion, however, is the burden that a person would experience in striving for the purpose of life, not the burden associated with the means to prolong life.

Severe pain, or great expenses causing the loss of other more important values, may result in the decision that one would have a difficult time striving for the purpose of life. On the other hand, the means to prolong life may not involve great pain, or expense, but prolonging life might still result in a grave burden in pursuing the purpose of life. For example, if one has a fatal pathology, there may be a comparatively painless method to circumvent its effects, yet one is not morally obliged to use that therapy if one believes it would be spiritually more beneficial to die now rather than later. A competent person with cancer who has contracted a severe case of pneumonia, for example, may determine that it is spiritually better to die of the pneumonia rather than wait and die a painful death from cancer. Thus, he or she may decide to forego the comparatively painless therapy needed to overcome the pneumonia.

Proxy Decisions

Even more difficult problems are involved when a decision based on grave burden must be made for another person. For example, if the life of an infant with a fatal pathology could be prolonged with some hope that the infant would develop cognitive-affective function, but if prolonging life would involve great pain, expense, or inhuman living conditions, is there always an ethical obligation to attempt to remove the pathology or arrest its effects? The federal regulations concerning care of debilitated infants indicate that this is required legally. Ethically speaking, however, if a fatal pathology is present, must a family consent to life-prolonging therapy for an infant who has severe genetic disease such as Lesch-Nyhan syndrome, or who will require nursing care 24 hours a day for the rest of his or her life? Should all children born with severe immunological deficiencies be raised in plastic bubbles, as was Baby David in Houston? In the case of Baby David, the means to prolong life were not painful, but after a time his life became severely burdensome. Again, we are called on to assess the burden of prolonged life, not the burden intrinsic to the means to prolong life. Even though the means to prolong life may be judged inexpensive or painless, using them may subject another human being to a life that is burdensome.

When making decisions for others, the proxy must realize that persons with impaired physiological function, even if their cognitive-affective function is weak, can still pursue the purpose of life. Thus, simply because an infant is debilitated does not imply automatically that he or she can be allowed to die from an existing fatal pathology. Moreover, a fatal pathology should never be induced in debilitated infants. On the other hand, the notion that there is an ethical obligation to prolong the life of every infant with a fatal pathology simply because prolonging life is possible is not ethically justifiable. Prolonging life may result in a grave burden for the infant in pursuing the purpose of life. Thus, when determining whether to seek to remove or circumvent a fatal pathology in a newborn infant or for an adult who is not competent, personal, familial, and social factors must be taken into account, as they are when one makes a decision for oneself.

Comfort Care

Maintaining that the life of a person need not be prolonged when a fatal pathology is present does not mean that the person should be neglected. Every dying person should be given spiritual and physical care. The ethical obligation to keep dying patients comfortable leads some to demand artificial hydration and nutrition for all patients, even those who are in an irreversible coma. But is there any medical indication that persons in this condition feel pain? Does the description of the effects of removing tube feeding given in the *Brophy* case apply to patients in an irreversible coma? Or is it a description more fitting for healthy individuals? In some hospices and infirmaries of religious institutes, the latter institutions being the embodiment of compassionate care for the dying, artificial hydration and nutrition are not used once a dying patient lapses into coma. In sum, evidence seems to be lacking that removing or withholding tube feeding from individuals in deep coma induces great pain or a new cause of death.

Conclusion

The significant ethical question in preserving our own life or the life of another person is "Does an ethical obligation exist to prolong life?" not "Are we able to prolong life?" Although inducing the pathology that causes death in an innocent person is never ethical, allowing a fatal pathology to take its normal course, not seeking to remove it or circumvent its effects, in some circumstances may be the better way to enable oneself or another person to pursue the purpose of life.

1. American Medical Association, Council on Ethical and Judicial Affairs, "Treatment of Patients in Irreversible Coma," March 15, 1986.
2. *Patricia E. Brophy vs. New England Sinai Hosptial, Inc.,* The Trial Court; Norfolk, MA; N.85E0009-G1.
3. National Conference of Catholic Bishops' Committee for Pro-Life Activities, "The Rights of the Terminally Ill" (July 2, 1986), *Origins* 16:12, Sept. 4, 1986, p. 222.

Ethical Issues in Joint Ventures   16

A joint venture, an agreement between a Catholic health-care organization and a healthcare organization that does not follow the *Ethical and Religious Directives for Catholic Health Facilities* to offer a service or conduct business concerned with healthcare, may involve several ethical issues. The Catholic healthcare organization that co-sponsors the joint venture may be a hospital, nursing home, or a corporation managing many hospitals. Some examples of joint ventures are office buildings jointly owned by Catholic hospitals and physicians, health maintenance organizations (HMOs) owned by Catholic health-care corporations, and insurance companies or businesses renting healthcare equipment and owned by Catholic healthcare corporations and independent businesspersons. A joint venture may be a not-for-profit or for-profit entity. In the latter case the profits accruing to the Catholic entity are to be used to benefit the not-for-profit sponsoring group. Thus, an office building may be a for-profit venture. Any profit accruing to the Catholic hospital that co-sponsors the office building must be devoted to the mission of the hospital.

In some instances of joint venture, the non-Catholic partner may not perform any services or actions that are contrary to Catholic teaching. In these cases, there are no direct ethical issues arising from the cooperation with the non-Catholic partner. In some cases, however, the non-Catholic partner of the joint venture may perform actions in other business ventures that are contrary to Catholic teaching or to sound morals. For example, the insurance company that joint ventures in an HMO program with Catholic hospitals may have other insurance policies that finance elective abortions or direct sterilizations. Although the Catholic HMO would not be allowed to fund elective abortions and sterilizations, the cooperation involved in the joint venture with the insurance company raises problems; association with it may be interpreted as approval of the activities of the insurance company. Another questionable joint venture would arise if the physicians who rent space in a professional building partly owned by a Catholic organization perform abortions at another hospital that is not Catholic.

Any time an individual Catholic or Catholic corporation cooperates with a person or corporation that performs actions contrary to Catholic teaching, the Catholic party must avoid formal cooperation in the prohibited action and must avoid giving scandal as well. Thus, the Catholic party in the joint venture must determine clearly that the prohibited actions of the partner in the joint venture are not a result of the joint venture. Moreover, to avoid scandal, the Catholic party should explain publicly that it rejects the unacceptable actions of the other partner and only tolerates the unapproved actions.

If we lived in a perfect world, there would be no need of joint ventures. But we live in a pluralistic society. Catholic healthcare facilities and corporations must cooperate in joint ventures to preserve their mission of healing in the name of Christ. When contemplating a joint venture, therefore, the first ethical question to ask is: Is the joint venture necessary to continue our apostolate? This question is overlooked by some organizations. Rather, they ask: "Will this joint venture make money?" or, "Will it result in more good than harm?" Profit of itself never justifies any work of the Christian apostolate. The joint venture should have some direct connection with the work of the apostolate. Some consultants representing large financial institutions encourage Catholic hospitals or healthcare coporations to joint venture in fast-food chains or parking lots to gain profits that will be directed to healthcare. The connection with apostolic activity seems tenuous.

The second ethical question concerned with joint ventures is: Does the partner in our joint venture perform actions in other ventures or businesses that are contrary to the teaching of the Church? The corporation co-sponsored by a Catholic organization should never engage in activities contrary to Church teaching. If the non-Catholic partner in the joint venture performs actions in other ventures or businesses that are contrary to Church teaching, then the Catholic corporation must ask: Are we sufficiently distancing ourself and the Church from the unacceptable actions of our partner performed in other areas? We cannot justify a joint venture by saying, "It does more good than evil." This might involve doing evil in order to achieve good. Rather, the work resulting from the joint venture must be morally acceptable. If evil actions are a concern, they must be clearly attributable to the other partner of the joint venture in an activity not associated with the joint venture involving the Catholic participant.

When forming joint ventures, as in many other issues in medical ethics, the principle of *double effect* is used. This principle has the four following conditions, with the last three really being a test to ensure the first condition is verified. To form a good conscience when an act is foreseen to have both beneficial and harmful consequences, the following conditions should be met:

1. The directly intended object of the act must not be intrinsically immoral

2. The intention of the agent must be to achieve the beneficial effects and to avoid the harmful effects as far as possible (i.e., must only indirectly intend the harm)

3. The foreseen beneficial effects must be equal to or greater than the foreseen harmful effects

4. The beneficial effects must follow from the action at least as immediately as the harmful effects. This principle is not easy to apply, but has been part of traditional Catholic teaching for centuries.

How does a Catholic healthcare institution or corporation make sure that it does not give scandal and does not actively support evil actions of a partner in a joint venture? Provided a true need exists for the joint venture to continue the good work of the Catholic entity, and provided that the joint venture does not perform any prohibited actions, the Catholic entity may find several ways to distance itself from the unacceptable activity of its partner. In an HMO, for example, the Catholic healthcare corporation will state publicly in the contract that it will not perform elective abortions or direct sterilizations and that it will not accept income resulting from these procedures if financed in other hospitals under the joint-venture HMO. In addition, the Catholic partner should retain the right to monitor advertising of the HMO.

To avoid even the semblance of approval of unacceptable practices, joint ventures which result in for-profit corporations should be avoided. Association with for-profit joint ventures may weaken the not-for-profit motivation and reputation of the Catholic entity. The mission of Catholic healthcare is an altruistic mission; surplus moneys derived in the course of the mission must be used to improve service, not as profit to benefit investors. Nothing can weaken the mission of Catholic healthcare more quickly than a concentration on profit. Thus, any semblance of such concentration should be avoided.

Resources

1. Howard Waitzen et al., "Deciding Against Corporate Management of a State-Supported Academic Medical Center," *New England Journal of Medicine* 315:20, Nov. 13, 1983, p. 1,299-1305.
2. Kevin D. O'Rourke, "An Ethical Perspective on Investor-Owned Hospitals," *Frontiers of Health Service Management.* 1:1, September 1984, pp. 10–26.
3. "Integrating Catholic Values and Business Survival Strategies," interview with Michael Doody, *Health Progress,* April 1986, pp. 18–25.

Healthcare Funding: 17
The Critical Question

In the state of Oregon recently, a seven-year-old boy died of leukemia. Shortly before his death, state health officials refused public funds for a potentially life-prolonging bone marrow transplant. Later, in the same state, a young mother was refused public funding for a liver transplant. Both actions resulted from a new policy of state health officials to refuse funding for bone marrow, pancreas, heart, or liver transplants.[1]

The decisions in Oregon have been portrayed as a preview of the decisions that will soon be necessary by officials in other states and by officials representing the federal government. The economic decisions that limit the access to healthcare have ethical implications. People will live or die as a result of these decisions. With this in mind, a closer investigation of the decisions in Oregon is in order.

The Principles

Is there a general principle that will ensure an ethical distribution of public funds to those in need of healthcare? In Oregon, the painful decisions to withhold funds were based on the assumption that basic healthcare should be provided before advanced or experimental care. Thus, the state officials in Oregon pointed out that basic healthcare was being provided for 24,000 more low-income people without any increase of funds by reason of the new policy. Moreover, they stated that "1500 pregnant women will receive prenatal care with the same amount of money that would pay for 30 organ transplants."[2] Many commentators and editorial writers, applauding the wisdom and courage of the Oregon allotment policy, declared that Oregon should be a model for federal agencies faced with the same decisions. A consensus seems to be present in the public forum, therefore, that basic care for the most people possible should be the principle on which access to healthcare for lower-income people is determined.

The Oregon decisions occur at a time when many people

are searching for principles to regulate the amount of U.S. assets devoted to healthcare. Callahan maintains that a new norm for funding healthcare for the aging must be developed.[3] At present, the healthcare research and therapy in the United States seems to be directed toward keeping people alive as long as possible, no matter what degree of function they might retain. Callahan persuasively questions whether this is a realistic norm, given the limited resources of our society and the certainty of death. He suggests that a more valid norm would be to afford as many people as possible the opportunity to live a beneficial life. Making such a radical readjustment in healthcare planning would direct funds away from the aging toward the younger members of society. Callahan realizes that his idea is prophetic, stating that it will not be accepted until his grandchildren are adults.

Discussion

The policies initiated in Oregon give some guidance for the future. Moreover, Callahan's ideas, which are explained much more intelligently and compassionately in his book, must be considered as the issue of allotting funds for research and healthcare therapy is discussed. However, both in Oregon and in Callahan's discussion, a vital question has not been considered sufficiently. At present, are we devoting a fair share of national assets to healthcare for low-income people? Although we may posit limited resources for healthcare, have we reached the reasonable limits of our resources? For the past 15 years, the proportion of our gross national product (GNP) devoted to healthcare has been a prominent discussion topic. Although healthcare is a significant percentage of the GNP, studies indicate that the citizens of our country devote significant monies to items that can only be deemed ephemeral. Are there many goods included in the GNP which are more important than access to healthcare? Moreover, is it that simple to distinguish between basic and advanced healthcare? If the criterion for distinguishing between basic and advanced healthcare is the success of the procedure, then some types of organ transplant currently may be designated as basic care, and other types will soon be in that category.

A prominent healthcare economist, Uwe Reinhardt, pointed out that Americans are delighted when figures indicate that the automobile industry is flourishing because this "is good for the economy and good for the country."[4] He asks whether the same attitude is not fitting in regard to healthcare. Although we do not want to foster a laissez faire attitude toward healthcare costs, we must admit Reinhardt is right in one regard. If we compare present and past percentages of the GNP devoted to healthcare, we are comparing apples to oranges. Medicine still has the same goals it had 40 years ago, but the means and methods of reaching these goals have changed significantly.

Conclusion

The great Swiss theologian, Karl Barth, said that a society must be judged on its willingness to care for its weak and impoverished members. Healthcare procedures should be evaluated carefully for cost efficiency, and the function of a patient should be considered when evaluating the effectiveness of healthcare procedures. It seems equally important, however, to evaluate whether or not the states and the federal government at present are devoting enough of our assets to offering access to healthcare for lower-income people.

1. Gilbert Welch and Eric Larson, "Dealing with Limited Resources: The Oregon Decision to Curtail Funding for Organ Transplantation," *New England Journal of Medicine,* July 21, 1988, pp. 171–173.
2. Welch and Larson.
3. Daniel Callahan, *Setting Limits: Medical Goals in an Aging*

Society, Simon & Schuster, New York, 1987.

4. Uwe Reinhardt, "Perspectives from an Economist", *Health Affairs Supplement*, 1988, pp. 96-104.

Development of Church   18
Teaching on Prolonging Life

The issue of when to prolong life and when to allow to die is debated acridly in our courts, hospitals, and homes. A study of the history and theology of the Catholic teaching on this issue may help to develop a consensus among those who accept the teaching of the Church, as well as among those who primarily follow the ethical norms of our pluralistic society.

The Purpose of Human Life

God gave us the gift of human life to show forth his goodness and love (Gn 1). We, in turn, show our love for God by respecting and fostering that gift of human life. Although we are called to life beyond human life, we do not disdain the gift of human life or reject it to hasten our advance toward eternal life (Lk 8:11).

As Jesus taught, love for God leads us not only to love ourselves, but to love others as well (Mt 22:37). One way to show our love for God, for ourselves, and for others is to prolong human life. Thus it is not an act of responsible human love to willfully and directly end one's own life or the life of another. Suicide and euthanasia have always been denounced by Christians because these acts are considered to be a serious violation of love for God.

Although human life is a great gift upon which many other goods depend, Sacred Scripture indicates it is not the supreme gift.[1] At times, the choice of another good may justify the indirect surrender of human life. In these circumstances, one does not choose death, but allows death to ensue because another greater good is chosen directly. Jesus on the cross, for example, freely gave his human life for the salvation of the world. Martyrs surrender their lives rather than deny God in their hour of crisis. Thus Christians have always maintained that life could be surrendered indirectly, if continuing to live would impede the response of love to God.

Human life, then, is a relative good in regard to the

absolute precept of Jesus: "Love God, and love your neighbor as yourself." Although prolonging life is usually a value because living humanly draws us closer to God, on some occasions prolonging life becomes an impediment or obstacle to returning God's love.

Teaching of Theologians

From the earliest centuries of the Church, when discussing acts that are opposed to care for life as an act of love for God, theologians focused on murder, suicide, and euthanasia, which by act or omission were intended to cause death directly.

But as the possibility of prolonging life through medicine or surgery increased, theologians started questioning how much effort one should expend to stay alive. Would it be a sin to reject efforts to prolong life if those efforts involved grave suffering, prohibitive expenses, or other serious burdens? Are there situations when choosing to avoid pain, suffering, or economic burden would bring about death only indirectly? In the sixteenth century, theologians began to discuss the questions: When would it not be suicide to allow oneself to die? When would it not be euthanasia to allow another to die?

The first explicit discussion of these questions is by Francisco di Vittoria, a Spanish Dominican theologian whose *Relectiones Theologicae* were originally published in 1557, 10 years after his death. In this work, Vittoria considered the moral obligation to use food to prolong life. He declared:

> If a sick man can take food or nourishment with a certain hope of life, he is required to take food as he would be required to give it to one who is sick. However, if the depression of spirits is so severe and there is present grave consternation in the appetitive power so that only with the greatest effort and as though through torture can the sick man take food, this is to be reckoned as an impossibility and therefore, he is excused, at least from mortal sin.[2]

Notice that Vittoria does not say a person in good health may starve himself because he is tired of living. Nor does he allow much leeway if the means (food) are effective ("a certain hope of life") and do not involve a grave burden. But he suggests that if a person is so sick and depressed that eating may become a grave burden, that person does not sin by not eating. Clearly, Vittoria recognizes psychic as well as physiological illness, and his notion of grave burden involves more than physical pain.

Vittoria also discusses the morality of using artificial means, namely drugs, to prolong life: "If one has moral certitude that drugs would heal and prolong life, then one should take the drugs himself or give them to a sick neighbor. If he does not, he would not be excused from mortal sin. But because a cure can seldom be certain, one need not utilize drugs even though very ill."

In considering the lawfulness of abstaining from specific foods, even if death would result, Vittoria maintained:

> It is one thing not to protect life and it is another not to destroy it. One is not held to protect his life as much as he can. Thus one is not held to use foods which are the best or most expensive even though those foods are the most healthful. Just as one is not held to live in the most healthful place neither must one use the most healthful foods. If one uses food which men commonly use and in quantity which customarily suffices for the preservation of strength, even though one's life is shortened considerably, one would not sin. One is not held to employ all means to conserve life but it is sufficient to employ the means which are intended for this purpose and which are congruous.[3]

To modern minds, Vittoria may seem liberal in the freedom he allows to refuse certain types of food even if death will ensue more quickly. But he wrote in a time when many would do penance by avoiding certain "more delicate" foods that might have been more healthful. For example, members of some religious orders would never eat meat. Moreover, the underlying reason for allowing people to abstain from healthful foods or to refrain from moving to a more healthful place was the choice of one good (e.g., penance or family stability) that rendered the other good onerous (e.g., eating meat or moving to the mountains). This "choice of goods" theory is basic to the Catholic tradition on prolonging life.

Ethical Norms

Several norms set out by Vittoria are operative in Catholic teaching today:

1. A moral obligation to prolong life was assumed, but it did not hold in all circumstances. Vittoria sought to be more specific about this obligation by asking (a) What means should be used to prolong life when one is not ill? and (b) What means should be taken to prolong life when one suffers from a fatal disease?

2. A means to prolong life need not be used if it is ineffective, if its effect is doubtful, or if it involves a grave burden for the person in question. To be judged effective, a medicine or procedure had to prolong life for a "significant length of time." A means could be effective and, at the same time, involve a grave burden to the patient—for example, eating expensive food or moving to a more healthful climate.

3. Artificial and natural means to prolong life should be evaluated according to the same principles: Will the means be effective, or will they cause a grave burden?

4. The burden or inconvenience involved in prolonging life includes the psychic and economic burden as well as the physical burden.

Ordinary and Extraordinary Means

The writing of Vittoria had great influence on many theologians who lived after him.[4] However, those theologians perfected Vittoria's thoughts by considering other cases in the light of contemporary medicine. For example, the introduction of anesthesia in the nineteenth century caused theologians to reconsider pain as a reason for refusing surgery. However, they were not called on to solve cases resulting from sophisticated methods of prolonging life. They did not discuss, for example, the obligation to prolong the life of a person in a coma because no effective means existed to do so. Therefore the distinctions of the past must often be made more exact.

The most important distinction in need of clarification is the one between the terms "ordinary" and "extraordinary" means to prolong life. These terms were gradually introduced in Catholic teaching over the centuries, although they were used with different meanings.[5] This led to confusion, which was noted in the document *Declaration on Euthanasia* published by the Vatican in 1980.[6] The confusion arises from the fact that originally the term "ordinary" was used in a generic sense to denote "common" means to prolong life, that is, means readily at hand and available to all. The term "extraordinary" originally referred to means that were either expensive, difficult to obtain, or inconvenient to arrange for the average person.

Over the years, the terms also were used in a specific ethical sense to signify whether a particular means to prolong life was morally obligatory (ordinary) or morally optional (extraordinary), for a particular person. Used in the generic sense, the terms signified whether the medicine or procedure in question was readily available for the average person. Used in the specific sense, the terms denoted whether the means to prolong life would be effective and without grave burden for a particular person.

In theological writings, the terms "ordinary means" and "extraordinary means" were often used interchangeably. A medicine or surgical procedure could be designated as ordinary in a generic sense but as extraordinary when applied to a particular patient. The noted medical-moral theologian Rev. Gerald Kelly, SJ, used the terms in this sense as late as 1950 when discussing the use of artificial hydration and nutrition.[7] After declaring that intravenous feeding is an "ordinary means" to prolong life, he stated that it could be considered extraordinary for a particular patient if he or she is not profiting spiritually from it.

Consideration of Circumstances

Pope Pius XII solved the ambiguous use of the terms ordinary and extraordinary when he stated that the determination of ordinary and extraordinary means requires a consideration of the "circumstances of persons, places, times, and cultures."[8] In using these terms, then, one should specify whether one is offering a general description of availability or a specific ethical judgment based on effectiveness or grave burden for a particular patient. Simply because a procedure is available does not imply that one has a moral obligation to use it. Respirators and blood transfusions are readily available in all acute care hospitals, but the hospitalized person has a choice about using them; this choice would require the patient to ask, Are these means effective? Would their use involve a grave burden?

A more modern complication concerning the terms ordinary and extraordinary means arises from the use of the terms in a medical context. In this context, the terms are used to distinguish medical therapy which is standard and accepted from medical therapy which is innovative or experimental. Thus antibiotics are ordinary therapy for pneumonia. But the artificial heart is extraordinary therapy for degenerative heart disease. When used in this sense, therapy which is extraordinary may become ordinary. Hence, the use of the terms ordinary and extraordinary means to prolong life always require further specification. The terms signify specific moral judgments only when considering the effectiveness or burden of a particular therapy for a particular person.

Why did the theologians who developed this teaching in regard to allowing to die fail to distinguish clearly between the generic (availability) and specific (moral obligation) use of these terms? Perhaps they presumed that most of the means to prolong life that were effective and readily available did not involve a grave burden for the person in question. As medical practice and technology became more advanced, however, many available and effective means to prolong life would result in a grave burden. For example, after the introduction of ether, amputations could be performed without severe pain, but a person might determine that living without two legs would be a grave burden and choose to live as long as possible without the amputation.

In summary, the theologians who wrote from the sixteenth to the nineteenth centuries considered morally obligatory (ordinary in the ethical sense) those means to prolong life which for a particular person would be effective in prolonging human life for a significant time and would not involve a grave inconvenience. They considered optional those means which for a particular person would be doubtfully effective for prolonging life or which would not prolong life for a significant length of time or would be judged too burdensome.

Significant Assumptions

To understand the teaching of the theologians and later statements of the Magisterium in regard to prolonging life and allowing to die, certain assumptions of the theologians' writings must be considered.

The theologians always assumed that suicide and euthanasia were moral evils. Both involve a direct intention of death and action (or inaction) from which death results directly. Clearly, the theologians did not conceive that they were fostering a direct choice of death when they stated that life need not be prolonged if the means are ineffective or involve a grave burden. Rather, they sought to allow the choice of a moral good for the person that may also lead indirectly to death.

For example, a person who would refuse an amputation without anesthesia because it would be too painful would be choosing to avoid excruciating suffering, even though the choice might hasten death. To say that Catholic teaching does not allow actions that indirectly bring about death or that may hasten death is erroneous.

The theologians of the past were applying the principle of double effect to the question of prolonging life. This principle is used extensively in Catholic theology but is not derived from faith.[9] Rather, the principle of double effect is derived from human experience and deals with undesirable effects of human choices; effects that may be foreseen as results of a choice but are not directly intended. If one fails to understand the principle of double effect, one will not be able to understand the difference between the acts of suicide or euthanasia and the act of allowing to die. It seems the dissenting judges in the *Brophy* case did not understand this principle—hence their impassioned statements concerning the majority opinion.[10] The majority opinion in the *Brophy* case acknowledged this principle implicitly when it stated that Brophy's proxy could choose a good—cessation of a degrading form of existence—even though death would result indirectly.[11] As Rev. Thomas O'Donnell, SJ, indicates, when artificial nutrition and hydration are withdrawn from a permanently comatose patient with an irreversible disease, the withdrawal of medical care is not the cause of death. "The cause of death is the irreversible disease, which has caused both the terminal coma and the inability to eat and drink. . . . Thus, rather than causing death, their withdrawal accurately could be viewed as letting inchoative death occur."[12] It seems that the courts faced with decisions concerning the maintenance or withdrawal of life support would do better to use the principle of double effect than to use ambiguous language such as "right to privacy," "right to die," or "death with dignity."

Decisions of Conscience

The theologians developing the Catholic tradition in regard to prolonging life did not seek to remove decisions of conscience from ailing individuals. Thus they did not compile a list of "objective means" that were too painful, expensive, difficult, or embarrassing for everyone. Neither did they seek to determine what would constitute "a significant length of time" to prolong life. Rather, they determined some generic reasons that would justify the choice of a good that indirectly led to death and called upon people to make the required specific applications. As befits sound theology, they set boundaries and allowed people freedom to make decisions within those boundaries.

The theologians sought merely to outline general actions that people in normal circumstances would avoid or perform to prolong life. But in regard to specific actions that might or might not be judged ineffective or too burdensome, they called on individuals to decide for themselves. Even eating food, as Vittoria pointed out, could be a "certain torture" for some depressed persons, and thus it would not be a morally obligatory means of prolonging life for the person in question. If, in some circumstances, eating food is a morally optional means to prolong life, how much more so might contemporary means to prolong life—ventilators, antibiotics, blood transfusions, and artificial nutrition and hydration—be judged optional if a sick person determines that the use of such procedures would be doubtfully effective or involve a grave burden?

Role of the Proxy

The Church's traditional teaching, then, calls on the individual to decide what is ineffective, what constitutes "a significant time," and what is too burdensome. The theologians presumed that if one is unable to decide for oneself, a relative or friend should decide. This is called "proxy consent" or "substitute judgment." Persons close to the one needing help are presumed to be moral agents for the incompetent person because they love the patient and will determine what is of benefit to the patient. If this presumption is proven false, others, even the courts, should make the ethical decisions for incompetent patients.

The Church's teaching does not impose on the proxy (or the courts) the incompetent person's wishes as the absolute norm for decision making. Pope Pius XII stated: "The rights and duties of the family depend upon the presumed will of the unconscious patient if he is of age and *sui juris* [having full legal right or capacity]. Where proper and independent duty of the family is concerned, they usually are bound only to use ordinary means."[13]

Thus the proxy should determine what is best for the patient, using the known wishes of the patient as a guide, but also considering the present circumstances. An incompetent person may have made known that a particular course of action be followed, but circumstances may have so changed that the proxy believes the incompetent patient would judge differently were he or she able to do so. For example, a person may have declared that given a certain physiological condition or disease, that all life support should be removed. But the proxy might determine to continue therapy in order to have the family gather before death, to alleviate pain, or to restore consciousness for spiritual purposes. The proxy should never carry out unethical actions, for example, acts constituting euthanasia, even if this is a known wish of the incompetent person. If the patient's wishes are not known, the proxy should consider what would be reasonable care for this patient. When determining "reasonableness," the proxy may ask, How will the decision for care affect other members of the family? The Church's teaching on proxy consent differs from the statements (although not always the practice) of some courts and certainly differs from the thought of many contemporary ethicists who use the person's autonomy as the absolute criterion for proxy decision making. Some contemporary ethicists would approve abetting suicide or mercy killing if it were clear this is "what the patient desired."

Spiritual Goal of Life

Gary M. Atkinson, PhD, points out that Vittoria and the other theologians were influenced by St. Thomas Aquinas, who explained that the moral measure of all human activity is whether it leads to God, the final end.[14] Thus, when the theologians described something as "too difficult," they implied that it would make loving God too difficult. The theologians did not emphasize this norm for judging what makes a means of prolonging life "too difficult." But Pope Pius XII, in 1957, clarified the tradition by explicitly presenting the spiritual goal of life as the norm for judging whether a grave burden is present. He declared:

> Normally [when prolonging life] one is held to use only ordinary means— according to the circumstances of persons, places, times, and cultures—that is to say, means that do not involve any grave burdens for oneself or another. A more strict obligation would be too burdensome for most people and would render the attainment of a higher, more important good too difficult. Life, health, all temporal activities are in fact subordinated to spiritual ends. On the other hand, one is not forbidden to take more than the strictly necessary steps to preserve life and health, as long as he does not fail in some more serious duty.[15]

Hence any medical therapy that would make the attainment of the spiritual goal of life less secure or seriously difficult could be judged a grave burden and could be considered an optional or extraordinary means to prolong life.

Emphasizing the spiritual goal of human life specifies more clearly the terms "ordinary" and "extraordinary," a specification that was not required when life-support systems were not as advanced as they are today. Contemporary life-support systems may prolong a state of existence which not only involves grave burdens for the patient, but also precludes spiritual activity on the part of the patient. Thus a more adequate and contemporary explanation of "ordinary" means to prolong life would be: those means which are obligatory because they enable a person to strive for the spiritual purpose of life without grave burden. "Extraordinary" means would seem to be: those means which are optional because they are ineffective or a grave burden in helping a person strive for the spiritual purpose of life. One cannot judge what is effective or a grave burden without considering the physiological condition, as well as the social and spiritual circumstances of the patient.

If it is reasonably certain that only physiological function can be prolonged in a comatose person, and that the human organ (the cerebral cortex), which is necessary for human spiritual activity, is unable to function, is there a moral obligation to prolong life? To pursue the spiritual purpose of life, one needs a minimal degree of cognitive-affective function. Therefore, if this function in an adult cannot be restored or if an infant will never develop this function, and if a fatal disease is present, it seems the adult or infant may be allowed to die because medical therapy is ineffective. Prolonging life simply because physiological function can be prolonged long after cognitive-affective function ceases irreparably is not a sufficient reason to continue therapy. Declaring medical therapy to be ineffective when spiritual function cannot be restored seems to be the ethical responsibility of physicians.[16]

People may define the spiritual goal of life in different ways. The phrase "loving God and neighbor" seems to express the Catholic tradition. Others would define the spiritual purpose of life as serving God and neighbor, leading a good life, enjoying life, relating to others, or contributing to society. No matter how the spiritual purpose of life is defined, some degree of cognitive-affective function is required to strive for it. If cognitive-affective function is irreparably lost, mere physiological function need not be prolonged because such therapy is ineffective to achieve the spiritual purpose of life.

Comfort Care

Maintaining that the life of a fatally ill person need not be prolonged does not imply that the person should be neglected. Every dying person should be given spiritual and physical care. A person whose spiritual function is irreparably lost is still a human being. We have a moral obligation to keep such patients comfortable. In regard to patients who may experience pain, the teaching of the Church (once again utilizing the principle of double effect) is quite clear. After declaring that physical suffering is unavoidable and that some Christians may choose to join their suffering with the sufferings of Christ, the Church states:

> Nevertheless it would be imprudent to impose a heroic way of acting as a general rule. On the contrary, human and Christian prudence suggest for the majority of sick people the use of medicines capable of alleviating or suppressing pain, even though these may cause as a secondary effect semiconsciousness and reduced lucidity. As for those who are not in a state to express themselves, one can reasonably presume that they wish to take these painkillers, and have them administered according to the doctor's advice. . . . In this case, of course, death is in no way intended or sought even if the risk of it is reasonably taken; the intention is simply to relieve pain effectively, using for this purpose painkillers available to medicine.[17]

The obligation to keep patients comfortable leads some to demand artificial hydration and nutrition for all patients in order to avoid physical suffering, even for those persons who are in an irreversible coma.[18] But is there any medical indication that persons in this condition feel physical pain? The neurological experts consulted in the *Brophy* case did not think so.[19] Moreover, in hospices and infirmaries of religious sisters, the latter institutions being the embodiment of compassionate care for the dying, artificial hydration and nutrition are seldom used once a dying patient lapses into a coma. In sum, evidence seems to be lacking that removing or withholding tube feeding from individuals in a deep coma or a persistent vegetative state results in great pain for the patient.

Burden to Others

Another latent issue in the traditional teaching of the theologians is the burden that caregivers, usually the family, might experience if a person's life is prolonged. If all circumstances must be considered, then the patient must ask, What will a decision to prolong my life mean to the people who must care for me? Would the burden be in accord with "the common sense of the Christian community" if the family would have to give the patient nursing care 24 hours a day and devote all its savings and income to that care?

Such problems are encountered often by families with severely debilitated newborn infants. Should the life of every newborn infant be prolonged, simply because it can be, regardless of the burdens this would cause the family?[20] About 20 years ago Baby David was born in Houston with severe combined immune deficiency (SCID). His life was prolonged by placing him in a germ-free plastic bubble for 13 years.[21] Ultimately, he said it was too difficult to live in that manner and he asked that the bubble be removed. He died shortly thereafter. The lives of other infants born with SCID could be prolonged in the same manner, but is this humane treatment? This significant question is not, Is it possible to prolong life? but rather, Is there an ethical obligation to prolong life?

Confirming the Traditional Teaching

In 1980 the Church Magisterium spoke again on the matter of prolonging life.[22] The document did not change the traditional teaching in any way, but sought to clarify it by stating:

1. The terms "ordinary" and "extraordinary" are less clear today; therefore the terms "proportionate" and "disproportionate" means might be more accurate.

2. The patient is to make the decision concerning proper care by studying the type of treatment to be used, its degree of complexity or risk, its cost, the possibilities of using it, and the results that can be expected, taking into account his or her condition and physical and moral resources. If the patient cannot speak for himself or herself, the family and the physician are to make the decision for proper care.

3. Experimental therapy even though risky may be used to

obtain knowledge for the treatment of future patients.

4. Only normal means, that is, means that do not carry a risk or a burden or are disproportionate to the results expected, may be used to prolong life. Such a choice is not suicide but rather accepting the human condition.

5. When death is imminent, therapy may be refused if it offers only a precarious and burdensome prolongation of life, but at the same time, the patient should be made comfortable.

Although the terms "proportionate" and "disproportionate," as well as the terms "burden" and "benefit," have replaced "ordinary" and "extraordinary" to a great extent, these more contemporary forms are not without potential ambiguity. Before determining whether a particular substance (whether natural or artificial) or medical therapy is proportionate or disproportionate, we must first determine the condition of the patient and whether the act or medical therapy in question is effective in prolonging life for a significant time or whether it involves a grave burden for a particular person. If these basic moral specifications are not discerned, then a consequentialist's interpretation could result from use of the new terms.

Norms Governing the Decision

In summary, then, these are the important norms in regard to prolonging life gathered from the theologians and the Magisterium:

1. Because human life is a great good, a presumption exists that human life should be prolonged. However, this presumption ceases if the means to prolong life are ineffective or involve a grave burden for a particular person.

2. The spiritual goal of life indicates when life-prolonging efforts become "ineffective" and enables one to measure grave burden.

3. No list of human actions or medical procedures can be determined as ordinary or extraordinary from a specific ethical perspective. A general description of means that are usually available, often prolong life, or seldom involve a grave burden is possible, but specific ethical judgments require a consideration

of all circumstances. Therefore one must specify whether the terms "ordinary" or "extraordinary" are being used in a general or specific sense.

4. When determining the moral obligation of whether to prolong life, we must know the patient's diagnosis and prognosis, as well as the "circumstances of persons, places, times, and cultures." Only then may one determine what is morally obligatory and what is optional.

5. If possible, the patient should be allowed to make decisions for himself or herself. If the patient is clearly not competent, however, a proxy is called. The proxy determines what is beneficial for the patient, taking into consideration all circumstances that a reasonable person would have considered, including the burdens on the family.

6. The decision to choose a good which entails discontinuing the use of a life-support system may hasten death. But death is the indirect result and occurs because one chooses another legitimate good.

Public Policy and Ethics

Although the ethics of personal decision making that will ensure the fulfillment of our response to God's love is a serious concern of the Church, the Church is also concerned with public policy in regard to prolonging life. Laws and court decisions are an important adjunct to personal decision making because they serve as an educational as well as a coercive factor in the lives of individuals.

When offering prudential advice to the courts and legislatures in regard to public policy, however, the statements of Church agencies should be in accord with the traditional teaching of the Church. A good example of accurate advice was offered by the National Conference of Catholic Bishops' Committee for Pro-Life Activities. In commenting on the statement on Uniform Rights of the Terminally Ill Act proposed by the Commission on Uniform State Laws, the bishops cautioned against promoting euthanasia and requested that legislation establish a strong presumption in favor of using artificial nutrition and hydration.

But the statement also allowed for withdrawal of life support that is ineffective or a grave burden and agreed that "laws dealing with medical treatment may have to take account of exceptional circumstances when even means for providing nourishment may become too ineffective or burdensome to be obligatory."[23]

Contrasted with the Pro-Life Committee's statement is the statement of the New Jersey State Catholic Conference in regard to the *Jobes* case. Nancy Ellen Jobes, 31 years old, was severely brain damaged and her existence was maintained by means of artificial nutrition and hydration in a nursing home. Her spouse asked the court for permission to withdraw all life-support systems. After maintaining that Nancy Jobes "is not dying," the *amicus curiae* brief of the New Jersey Catholic Conference stated: "The conference maintains that nutrition and hydration, being basic to human life, are aspects of normal care, which are not excessively burdensome, and should always be provided to a patient."[24] In June 1987, the New Jersey Supreme Court granted permission for the withdrawal of all life-support systems from Mrs. Jobes stating that the right of a patient to refuse life-sustaining medical treatment may be exercised by the patient's family or close friend. Thus the court held that in certain circumstances withdrawal of nutrition and hydration is neither euthanasia nor suicide.

Although the intent of the New Jersey Catholic Conference to avoid "a slippery slope" in matters of allowing to die is laudable, accurate ethical distinction must be used or the Church teaching in the matter, which has been respected and followed by many in our pluralistic society, will lose credibility.

Conclusion

Understanding and following the Church teaching in regard to life support will not make the decision to withhold or withdraw medical therapy an easy one. Such decisions will always be accompanied by anxiety and sorrow. Decisions of proper ethical care will continue to bother and befuddle healthcare professionals, patients, and their families. Indeed, the degree of anxiety and sorrow accompanying these decisions may be a good measure of one's humanity. However, the Church teaching will enable people to make just and compassionate decisions that express effectively their love for God. The papal Magisterium in the latest statement in this regard sums up the issue well: "Life is a gift of God, and on the other hand death is unavoidable. . . . Death marks the end of our earthly existence but at the same time it opens the door to immortal life. Therefore, all must prepare themselves for the event in the light of human values, and Christians even more so in the light of faith."[25]

1. Patrick Senay, "Biblical Teaching on Life and Death," in *Moral Responsibility in Prolonging Life Decisions*, Donald McCarthy and Albert Moraczewski, eds., Pope John XXIII Medical-Moral Research and Education Center, St. Louis, 1981.
2. "Relectio IX; de Temperentia," *Relectiones Theologicia*, 1587: cf. Relecciones Teologicas, edition critica, Imprenta La Rafa, Madrid, 1933–35, Vol. III. The *Relectio* was a lecture that Vittoria, the preeminent theologian at the University of Salmanca, Spain, would give at the beginning of the school year. These lectures always treated a difficult, contemporary ethical issue. For example, he considered the rights of the natives in the New World, the rights of the Spanish to convert the natives, the norms for international law, and other timely topics. Hence, we may presume that in his time the question of prolonging life was as disputed as it is in our time.
3. "Relectio IX; de Temperentia."
4. Daniel Cronin, *The Moral Law in Regard to Ordinary and Extraordinary Means of Conserving Life*, Gregorian, Rome, 1958.

5. The use of the terms increased in the seventeenth century. D. Banez (1604) speaks about extraordinary means being optional. By the time of Cardinal de Lugo (1660), the terms "ordinary" and "extraordinary" are firmly in place.

6. Sacred Congregation for the Doctrine of the Faith, "Vatican Declaration on Euthanasia" (June 26, 1980), *Origins* 10:10, Aug. 14, 1980, pp.154–157.

7. Gerald Kelly, "The Duty to Preserve Life," *Theological Studies*, June 1950, p. 218.

8. Pope Pius XII, "The Prolongation of Life," *The Pope Speaks* 4:4 1958, p. 343; Sacred Congregation for the Doctrine of the Faith.

9. Joseph Mangan, "An Historical Analysis of the Principle of Double Effect," *Theological Studies*, 10, 1949, pp. 40–61; John Connery, "Catholic Ethics: Has the Norm for Rule Making Changed?" *Theological Studies*, June 1981, p. 232.

10. Leslie Rothenberg, "The Dissenting Opinions: Biting the Hand That Won't Feed," *Health Progress*, December 1986, p. 38.

11. *Patricia Brophy vs. New England Sinai Hospital, Inc.* (Mass. Sup. Jud. Ct., Sept. 11, 1986). "In certain thankfully rare circumstances the burden of maintaining the corporeal existence degrades the very humanity it was meant to serve. The law recognizes the individual's right to preserve his humanity, even if to preserve his humanity means to allow the natural processes of a disease or affliction to bring about death with dignity."

12. Thomas O'Donnell, SJ, "Comment," *Medical Moral Newsletter*, February 1987, p. 7.

13. Pope Pius XII.

14. Gary M. Atkinson, "Theological History of Catholic Teaching on Prolonging Life," in *Moral Responsibility in Prolonging Life Decisions*, Donald McCarthy and Albert Moraczewski,

eds., Pope John XXIII Medical-Moral Research and Education Center, St. Louis, 1981.

15. Pope Pius XII.

16. Edmund Pellegrino and David Thomasma, *For the Patient's Good*, Oxford Press, New York, 1988, p. 73.

17. Sacred Congregation for the Doctrine of the Faith.

18. New Jersey Catholic Conference Brief, "Providing Food and Fluids to Severely Brain Damaged Patients," *Origins*, Jan. 22, 1987, p. 582.

19. See note 11: "Testimony of American Society of Neuro-Surgeons," p. 12.

20. While the most recent regulations from the federal government concerning cure for debilitated infants may allow, through a generous interpretation, consideration of the burden to the parents, the first two sets of norms (which were later declared unconstitutional by federal courts) did not allow for consideration of this burden. Clearly, the interpretation of "grave burden" on the part of parents had led to the violation of rights on the part of some debilitated infants such as Baby Doe in Indiana, but rights are not protected and equitably decisions are not fostered by means of unethical laws and/or regulations. See *Federal Register*, July 5, 1983, "Nondiscrimination on the Basis of Handicap Relating to Health Care for Handicapped Infants," 45 CFR part 84, pp. 30846–30852; April 15, 1985, "Child Abuse and Neglect Prevention and Treatment Program," 45 CFR part 1340, pp. 14878–14901; Jan. 12, 1984, "Nondiscrimination on the Basis of Handicap; Procedures and Guidelines Relating to Health Care for Handicapped Infants; Final Rule," 45 CFR, pp. 1622–1655.

21. "David the 'Bubble Boy' and the Boundaries of the Human," *Journal of the American Medical Association*, Jan. 4, 1985, pp. 74–76.

22. Sacred Congregation for the Doctrine of the Faith.

23. National Conference of Catholic Bishops' Committee for

Pro-Life Activities, "The Rights of the Terminally Ill" (July 2, 1986), *Origins* 16:12, Sept. 4, 1986, p. 222.

24. New Jersey Catholic Conference Brief.
25. Sacred Congregation for the Doctrine of the Faith.

Ethical Issues in Research 19

Research is the lifeblood of medical progress. Ensuring ethical research programs, however, is not always easy. For example, after the heart of a baboon was implanted in an infant with hypoplastic left-sided heart syndrome, the procedure was criticized because scientific as well as ethical norms were not observed.[1] Specifically, the researchers "were far too optimistic about the therapeutic benefits." Moreover, the artificial heart program has been questioned on ethical grounds because benefits are described in less than accurate language.[2] One heart recipient, for example, described by the hospital as being in satisfactory condition, had three strokes, lost his power of speech and memory, and never achieved the quality of function predicted by the medical team.

The disconcerting aspect of both these cases is that they were approved by institutional review boards (IRBs) as being ethically acceptable. Although a full ethical analysis of these cases is not the purpose of this essay, it might be helpful to consider some basic ethical concepts that, if emphasized and underlined, might guide IRBs more surely.

Principles

Research programs in the United States receive their ethical direction from the norms published by the Department of Health and Human Service (DHHS). These norms are applied by IRBs, which function at every research institution.[3] The ethical norms of DHHS seem to be inadequate for two reasons:

1. The norms of DHHS do not distinguish between informed consent and proxy consent; thus, they allow decisions to be made for incompetent persons that do not respect their rights.

2. The norms of DHHS that apply only to children involve the distinction between therapeutic research (what will benefit a patient personally) and nontherapeutic research (what will benefit society by providing new knowledge but will not benefit the subject of the research protocol).

Let us say a word about these distinctions. To respect the

worth and integrity of an individual, informed consent is required before a person can be a subject of a research program. Informed consent means that the subject has knowledge concerning the research, understands how it will affect him or her, and freely consents to be in the program. Clearly, the only people capable of giving informed consent are those who are conscious and competent. If one is in a coma, a minor, senile, or retarded, one cannot give informed consent. If there is a question of admitting a person who is a minor, in a coma, senile, or retarded into a research program, then the guardian of that person must be consulted. The guardian, however, does not give informed consent for the minor. Rather, the parent or guardian gives *proxy consent*. When we give proxy consent for another, we act as benefactor for that person. We are allowed to give permission for only those procedures that would benefit the patient. In the same way that informed consent protects the worth and integrity of a competent person, so the principle of "only benefitting" a minor or ward protects the worth and integrity of a noncompetent person.

Research and Practice

The limits of proxy consent become even more evident when we emphasize the distinction between therapeutic and nontherapeutic research. Competent persons who offer informed consent are able to engage in research projects that do not offer therapeutic benefit but that will improve human knowledge. Thus, competent persons can take a risk with their own well-being, risking injury, anxiety, or impairment to benefit other human beings. However, one is not able to present another person with the risk of possible pain, injury, or impairment unless this is associated with therapy needed for the person in one's care. If one equates informed consent and proxy consent, then one gives to the person granting proxy consent the right to "use" other people for nontherapeutic research.

Discussion

The lack of clarity in regard to the nature and limits of consent and research may incline IRBs to approve protocols merely by asking the question, "Does the person giving consent know the risks and benefits?" But the questions, "Is this proxy consent?" or "Is this nontherapeutic research?" are often overlooked. Thus, a minor may be subject to harm or pain, or a competent person may not have the benefits and risks explained accurately.

The Nuremberg Declaration, a statement made to counteract the research atrocities perpetuated on helpless victims in World War II "who were going to die anyway," is very careful to limit the subjects of research projects. It states:

> The voluntary consent of the human subject is absolutely essential. This means that the person involved should have legal capacity to give consent; should be able to exercise free power of choice . . . and should have sufficient knowledge and comprehension . . . to enable him to make an understanding and enlightened decision."[4]

Some may reply to our considerations that children and other persons equal to minors should "wish to benefit others" and therefore should be included in nontherapeutic research. This is beside the point. To determine what others *should* wish is not the right given to proxies. Rather, they are given only the right to determine what would be of benefit to their wards. Some may wish to extend the term *benefit* to include social values. Thus, some would claim that the impaired or retarded persons and children do "benefit" from nontherapeutic research because they contribute to the common good. By using words metaphorically, one can justify anything. Benefit in the context of research implies that the research protocol will be therapeutic for the person who is the subject.

Finally, if we limit the research on infants and retarded and impaired people, even when these persons are competent, will it not slow down medical progress? For example, if we wait until there is a possibility of true benefit for an infant with hypoplastic heart syndrome before allowing infants into the research program, will we not slow down research on xenotransplants? If we insist on a more accurate description of benefits from the artificial heart, would we not impede medical progress? Yes, insisting on more rigorous ethical norms may slow down research, but there is a much more important value at stake than knowledge of xenotransplants or artificial hearts. The value we are concerned with is how we will care for the young, the weak, and the impaired persons in our society.

As the Helsinki Statement, another attempt of the international scientific community to establish ethical norms for research, declared: "In research on man the interest of science or society should never take precedence over consideration of the well-being of the subject."[5] In sum, the federal norms seem inadequate to the task of ensuring ethical research projects.

1. Arthur L. Caplan, "Ethical Issues Raised by Research Involving Xenografts,"*Journal of the American Medical Association*, Dec. 20, 1985.
2. "Jarvik Heart Ban Almost Urged," *St. Louis Post-Dispatch*, Feb. 21, 1986.
3. Federal Register, March 8, 1983 "Protection of Human Subjects," 45 CFR 46 p. 4–18.
4. Nuremberg Code, Nuremberg Military Tribunal, 1946, *Encyclopedia of Bioethics*, vol. 4, p. 1764.
5. Declaration of Helsinki, World Health Association, 1964 and 1975, *Encyclopedia of Bioethics*, vol. 4, p. 1769.

Role of Ethics Committees in   **20**
Medical Decision Making

One of the first empirical studies of ethics committees in hospitals found that ethics committees are used for everything from "acting as a public relations tool for justifying unpopular decisions resulting from discontinuing unprofitable services" to "serving as an alternative to the courts."[1] Although most ethics committees have a more limited purview, the study revealed that many ethics committees believe they should be involved at some time in particular medical decisions concerning patient care.

In this essay, basing considerations on the nature of the physician-patient relationship, we discuss the responsibility for ethical decision making in medicine. The discussion attempts to set forth realistic guidelines for the activities of ethics committees.

The Principles

Physicians promise to help patients to avoid illness, to regain health, or to live with infirmity as vitally as possible. The objectives of the physician-patient relationship always presuppose that the physician will offer help in accord with the patient's personal values. Thus, medicine is not an abstract science dealing only with scientific principles. Rather, medicine is an application of scientific principles to particular individuals. The social and spiritual dimensions of the persons to whom scientific principles are applied, as well as their varying desires and needs, make the inclusion of values a necessity in forming a medical plan. For this reason, Leon Kass maintains that medicine, by its very nature, is a "moral enterprise."[2]

In the recent past, some philosophers have maintained that in science one cannot progress logically from the "is" to the "ought," from the scientific to the ethical. Thus, they maintain, science and its applications are "value free"; the moral dimension of scientific and medical judgments is something added from other disciplines. If values are intrinsic to decisions concerning medical care, however, then there is no reason to say that a transition must be made from "is" to "ought." The "ought," or ethical dimension, is an integral part of the medical decision.

Physicians and patients (or proxies) both have something to contribute to the medical care decision. The patient or proxy primarily expresses the desires and values of the person seeking medical help. The physician mainly makes a diagnosis and designs a medical care program in accord with the expressed wishes of the patient. The medical care decision is a cooperative product based on mutual trust.

What role does medical ethics have in this description of medical decision making? Medical ethics is not a new subspecialty within medicine. Physicians, not ethicists or ethics committees, are responsible for ensuring that the ethical perspective is present in medical decisions. Maintaining that physicians decide one aspect of patient care and ethicists another is a caricature of both medicine and ethics. Ethicists are able to help physicians prepare for medical decision making in accord with the accepted ethical norms, but ethicists may never replace physicians. What are accepted ethical norms? Obtaining informed consent for therapy is an example of an accepted ethical norm for medical care. Ethicists help physicians understand the essential elements of informed consent, but physicians ensure that informed consent is obtained.

Another accepted ethical norm of medical care states that physicians should not induce death but may allow patients to die in certain circumstances. Helping physicians understand the circumstances that allow them to apply this important but subtle norm is the role of the ethicist. Although a body of knowledge exists that justifies calling medical ethics a distinct discipline, and thus justifies the role of medical ethicists, there is no reason to make the medical ethicist a principal participant in medical decision making. In general, the medical ethicist acts as an educator and, in specific cases, as a consultant, which is simply a more personal form of education.

If we are to preserve the integrity of the physician-patient relationship, the ethics committee should be envisioned as a group of persons fulfilling the role of the medical ethicist. Thus, they offer to healthcare professionals and their patients only education and consultation.

Discussion

With this somewhat more specified function assigned to medical ethics and ethics committees, several observations are in order:

1. Ethics committees should devote intense activity to self-education. If the committee is to sponsor education and consultation according to accepted ethical principles, then the committee must be knowledgeable about the principles in question. Common sense does not suffice for sound ethical decisions. The President's Commission for the Study of Ethical Problems in Medicine and Biomedical and Behavioral Research has developed some principles for our pluralistic society. The Catholic Church, in accord with its notion of the nature of the human person, has also developed ethical norms for medical care. Depending on the character of the healthcare facility, the ethics committee should school itself in one or both sets of these principles.

2. The membership of the ethics committee need not include people "from all walks of life." When stating regulations for ethics committees, there is a tendency to require membership of persons who are "nonscientific," who "represent the community," or who are "consumers of healthcare." Clearly, when membership of "outsiders" on ethics committees is recommended, there is a possibility that ethical decisions in medicine will be based on public opinion rather than on accepted ethical principles and the knowledge of medical practice. People from all walks of life may serve effectively on ethics committees in healthcare facilities if they are knowledgeable about ethics, but they do not qualify as ethical experts simply because they are "outside" the profession of healthcare. Rather, persons qualify for ethics committees through their ability to analyze issues from well-reasoned ethical perspectives.

3. The main purpose of ethics committees is to sponsor education programs for all persons associated with the health-

care facility. The formulation of policy in regard to ethical issues, such as policies for do-not-resuscitate (DNR) orders or transplantation of organs, simply represents more specific educational programs. If consultation on an ethical issue is requested by a physician or a patient (or proxy), the purpose should be to help the physician and/or patient to sort out their thinking. The ethics committee does not replace the physician or the patient. The concept that the ethics committee becomes some sort of jury before whom evidence is presented is a travesty of ethical decision making.

Conclusion

The foregoing vision of ethics committees does not call for a deemphasis of these committees. True, if the relationship between the physician and the patient is to be respected, ethics committees will have a more limited responsibility than some would desire. However, the need for education in medical ethics should not be underemphasized. Physicians and other health-care professionals do not know intuitively the principles of medical ethics. Thus, they require the input and expertise of the ethics committee in their ethical decision making.

1. Bernard Lo, "Behind Closed Doors: Promises and Pitfalls of Ethics Committees," *New England Journal of Medicine* 317:46, July 2, 1987 pp. 46-50.
2. Leon Kass, *Toward a More Natural Science*, Free Press, New York, 1985, p. 211.

Challenging Ethics Committees

Members of the ethics committee of Los Angeles County High-Desert Hospital in Lancaster, CA, were sued for $10 million in a malpractice suit filed on behalf of Elizabeth Bouvia, a quadraplegic, cerebral palsy victim. Her name has been equated with attempts to stop methods of artificial nutrition and to allow her to die, first in 1983, then in 1986.

The medical director of Los Angeles County High-Desert Hospital claimed that he had discussed the issue of whether or not to remove Bouvia's feeding tube with the members of the ethics committee in 1986. He stated that the members of the ethics committee were in agreement and that his actions were approved by and responsive to the committee's discussions. Significant confusion surrounds who is responsible for the decision that was made to maintain Bouvia's nasogastric feeding tube until a court ordered it removed. No clear record exists in the news of the actual deliberations of the ethics committee in this matter. Also, there is little to indicate that there are minutes of meetings in which the ethics committee did or did not make a case to continue or to withdraw the artificial feeding tube.

The issue of liability for decisions made or responsibility for decisions that could bring an entire ethics committee into the court system have been discussed by many people who have advocated the establishment of ethics committees in individual institutions.[1] What the *Bouvia* case and the lawsuit raise, however, are questions of whether or not institutional ethics committees (IECs) ought to be involved in medical decision making. If they are involved in medical decision making, what sort of liability or responsibility do the individual members of the ethics committee have for the decisions made? This question goes to the heart of the purpose of IECs. What is their proper function and goal? How should they be acting within the institution? What are the limits that should be placed upon them?

Functions and Goals of Institutional Ethics Committees

IECs have functions, which are not exclusive of one another. Also each function has to be tailored to the needs of the particular institution.

1. The first function reflects what might have happened in the *Bouvia* case. The IEC is a *decision maker*. Those who advocate that IECs should be decision makers claim that the committee can serve a useful purpose by gathering together a variety of people from different disciplines to reflect on a specific ethical issue when requested by the physician, patient, the patient's family, or some other provider within the institution. In a decision-making role, the conclusions of the committee are binding. Advocates of the decision-making function argue that difficult ethical issues require more than one discipline. In addition, some argue that such decision-making responsibilities for the IEC will alleviate difficult and vexing ethical decisions for the physician. The difficulty with such responsibilities for the IEC is that they can violate the primary ethical responsibilities of professionals.

If the IEC of Los Angeles County High-Desert Hospital did act as a decision-making body about the appropriateness of Bouvia's feeding tube, then the committee should be held accountable for the decision.

2. Tangentially related to the decision-making process is a *consultative function* for the IEC. In a consultative process, individuals knowledgeable about medicine, ethics, and patient values gather to provide an opportunity to sort through and discuss difficult concerns.

The consultative body balances a variety of ethical concerns. The first is the right of patients to make decisions for themselves in accordance with their particular values. The second involves values the institution upholds and wishes to continue to uphold in its delivery of healthcare. The third is the professional value of the person who delivers medical care. Finally, the consultative group may provide an opportunity for education and discussion that would not be available in another setting.

3. Another function for IECs is *education*. This is the broadest function; it requires the committee to educate itself, employees of the institution, the patients who seek services, their families, and the community. Education has a variety of goals. It can provide people with information relative to their own particular decision making, such as the various elements to consider when deciding upon a "do-not-resuscitate" order for oneself or for another. The IEC also can educate the institution and the surrounding community about the economic structures and difficulties present in healthcare. Education can raise issues about the allocation of resources, how much money should be spent, and what values people wish to realize when receiving healthcare services. The educational goal is the most significant goal of an ethics committee.

4. Finally, ethics committees can become involved in *policy interaction* or *policy deliberation*. An ethics committee can be a forum for the development of policies that cut across the medical staff, nursing staff, and administrative staff and have a direct effect on the values of individual patients. The IEC also can be used as a mechanism to review policies developed in other areas of the institution. Policies also may be initiated from the IEC if the committee membership is representative of the major professional bodies and managers of the institution.

Conclusion

Institutional ethics committees must decide what the appropriate function and goal of the committee will be within the institution. The IEC may decide to pursue only one function or may pursue more than one of the different objectives.

The difficulty with ethics committees pursuing a decision-making structure is evident in the *Bouvia* case. Taking the ethical decision away from the providers of medical care and placing it before a committee is unethical.

If ethics committees are consultative bodies, then a specific type of training for the committee is necessary. This is very different from the training necessary if only education or both education and policy interaction is the IEC's primary goal.

In short, whatever goals and objectives an IEC has within an institution, it is responsible and accountable for the activities, decisions, and the processes used to address the ethical issues and concerns of healthcare. Whether liability will scare people away from participating in IECs remains to be seen. If individuals are making medical decisions about treatment issues for patients, then they ought to be liable for mistakes in judgment or for inappropriate decisions. If IEC members are engaging in consultative, educational, and policy procedures, then they ought to be held accountable for those activities, but not liable for the decision made in the clinical setting.

1. Bowen Hosford, *Bioethics Committees,* Aspen Publications, Rockville, MD, 1986, pp. 307–319.

Cases and Articles Part III

AIDS: Three Sets of Ethical Issues 22

During the summer of 1981 an acquired immune deficiency syndrome caused by a human T lymphocyte-tropic retrovirus was recognized and reported in the United States and France. This new disease came to be known as AIDS. For those who suffer from the many opportunistic infections that arise as a result of a suppressed immune system, death results. There is no cure. Also, no vaccine is presently available to prevent one from contracting the virus.

The presence of AIDS in the United States has caused anxiety in almost every sector of the population. Many health-care workers and laboratory technicians fear they will contract the virus through their jobs. Parents fear for their children attending the same school as a child who has a positive test for the antibody but no symptoms of any opportunistic infections. Neighborhoods protest the presence of victims of this syndrome in nursing homes, hospitals, and other shelters. And there are the fears of those who are presently suffering from AIDS, those who know they have the antibody but have no symptoms, and those who suffer from AIDS-related complex (ARC). Some of these victims of AIDS have been abandoned by family and society and left to die alone.

Numerous ethical issues are involved in dealing with this new disease. Some of the issues are the result of ignorance and fear; some are complicated issues of treatment protocols and public policy. Confidentiality, knowledge about the presence of the antibody in one's body fluids, and the common good are some of the issues that must be examined carefully.

The first ethical problem is knowledge and truthfulness about the disease for the healthcare professional, for the victim of AIDS, and for the public. AIDS is not one of the most contagious diseases known and it is not transmitted through casual contact. Although those who suffer from full-blown AIDS die, usually within a relatively short time, it is not known whether all who have tested positive for the AIDS antibody will contract full-blown AIDS or whether some may live asymptomatically with the virus for life. The virus has been found in a variety of body fluids, but there is no evidence that contact with all these fluids transmits the virus. Intimate sexual contact and intravenous drug use, where one shares needles with another infected person, account for 90 percent of all cases in the United States. Blood transfusions, thanks to the development of accurate tests for the presence of the antibody to the virus, will seldom spread the virus.

AIDS is also present in other parts of the world. In some areas of the world it is more prevalent in the heterosexual population and other groups of people than in the at-risk groups that have been identified in the United States. Subsequently, it is not correct to say that AIDS is a homosexual disease or a drug user's disease. There are epidemiological reasons why these two groups are most affected in the United States, but AIDS must be seen in a larger context. Without accurate information, most of the other ethical problems are unresolvable.

The second cluster of ethical issues concerns victims of full-blown AIDS or ARC. Sometimes these people are shunned by healthcare professionals because of fear and ignorance. Should healthcare professionals treat or care for AIDS patients? Can they refuse to treat them on ethical or professional grounds? First, the specific pattern for the spread of the virus is not a part of medical practice. Second, since the illness is random, blaming the victim and refusing to treat a patient because of his or her illness as the result of supposed moral failure is unethical. Third, because of the severity of the illness, all full-blown AIDS patients die. Whether cure, care, or palliation is an appropriate goal for the AIDS victim will depend on the type of infection and how far the disease has progressed.

In all circumstances, however, the healthcare professional's purpose is to be of service to the sick. This service should be marked by compassion and care, regardless of the disease of the person. Because some facts about AIDS are not completely understood, there may be certain precautions which the healthcare professional should take, such as using an ambu bag for resuscitation and taking additional precautions when in contact with blood products and needles. However, these precautions are no reason for total isolation or abandonment of the patient.

The value and esteem of the medical profession does not require heroic life-giving measures of providers, but reasonable risk is involved in the treatment of any person with an infectious disease.

A third set of ethical issues involves public education and public policy. Education needs to be addressed at many levels. First is the issue of education for those who are known to have the AIDS antibody. In cases where screening is required, as in blood donations and soon in the military, what should be told to those who are found to have the antibody? Also, when should this be told: after the first ELISA test, or only after the more expensive Western Blot test? Who pays? What happens to the information? Can it be kept confidential? Can one be denied health insurance because of a positive test? Resolving these issues is difficult. Certain values should be remembered. Knowledge about one's health is crucial to making good decisions. For some, knowledge about whether or not the antibody exists provides assurance, whereas for others it will create anxiety. Can the fact that some are anxious prevent others from knowing test results? Can one educate society to the fact that the presence of the antibody may not mean one will develop full-blown AIDS? Can one stress the fact that, although one may not suffer from the virus, one can transmit it? This knowledge may be very important for one's sexual life and for one's reproductive decisions.

Second, the educational value is knowledge that will help to quell irrational fears. This could contribute to the dialogue necessary for good public policies in regard to children and schools, care for patients suffering from AIDS, and proper approaches to certain proposals such as closing bathhouses for gays or legally selling needles and syringes to intravenous drug abusers. Reasoned discussion within a public educational forum may prevent AIDS victims from being neglected and may help stop the transmission of the virus by stressing that the greater risk may come from infected people with no symptoms of the illness who spread the virus unwittingly.

Finally, education must encompass the traditional values of medical care and confidentiality. It should stress that ambiguity and uncertainty are always a part of the practice of medicine, and as research and work continue, greater knowledge will be obtained. To act out of fear because everything about AIDS is not known is to act irrationally. Rather, one must treat AIDS with the seriousness it deserves, the caution necessary to contain its transmission, and compassion for its victims that is easily given to others suffering from life-threatening illnesses. The seriousness of AIDS cannot countenance injustice.

Screening for AIDS: 23
Individual Liberty and Public Health

Circumstances surrounding the spread of acquired immune deficiency syndrome (AIDS) in the United States have intensified arguments over screening for the virus that causes the fatal illness.

Should anyone have to undergo screening? Should everyone? Who should pay for the testing? Should it make a difference whether the screening is voluntary or mandatory? Should results be shared with sexual partners, insurors, or anyone other than the person tested? How can AIDS patients' rights of privacy and autonomy be balanced against those of family, acquaintances, healthcare workers, and society in general?

Discussion of how to deal with a new, communicable and so far incurable illness would be highly charged under any circumstances. The fact that in the United States AIDS has spread primarily among homosexuals and intravenous drug abusers has boosted the level of emotion to an even higher plateau. Healthcare professionals, through institutional ethics committees (IECs), must take care to look at the facts objectively, assess the risks carefully, and participate in the discussion of AIDS screening from a rational rather than an emotional perspective.

The Facts

In the 1980s, the human immune deficiency virus (HIV), which causes AIDS, has spread rapidly. How many people are infected by HIV is not known. It is known that HIV is transmitted through blood and body fluids. The virus has been cultured in almost every bodily fluid, but not every bodily fluid is necessarily an avenue for transmitting it.

Currently, there is no way to predict how many people who test positive for HIV will suffer AIDS or AIDS-related complex (ARC), which causes a number of symptoms of full-blown AIDS. The simple and devastating fact is that exposure to HIV can result in AIDS, and AIDS is 100 percent fatal.

Although a vaccine or cure may be developed someday,

none is on the immediate horizon. No one has survived AIDS, but many people have lived for a long time after exposure to HIV without experiencing any of the medical complications common to AIDS patients. How long an HIV-positive individual can live before becoming ill—or whether a person can live a normal lifetime after exposure to HIV—is unknown.

The Fears

The facts about HIV and AIDS, and the recognition that so much is not known, cause great concern in public health circles, acute care hospitals, long term care facilities, schools, and neighborhoods. Although most AIDS cases so far can be traced to homosexual or bisexual activity, shared needles, and contaminated blood transfusions, HIV is moving insidiously into virtually every sector of American society. Its proportions have become epidemic, and fear of it has grown.

Misinformation causes confusion and unnecessary panic. Some would-be blood donors worry needlessly that they might contract AIDS by giving blood. Other people worry about the spread of HIV through casual contact in the classroom, on the playground, or in bathrooms, despite the almost nonexistent possibility of that happening. People who suffer from ARC or AIDS are concerned about whether they will receive proper medical attention. HIV carriers worry that society will shun them and insurance companies will drop them. Healthcare workers are concerned about balancing proper attention to AIDS patients against their own safety and health. Across society, many people are reassessing and changing their lifestyles in the areas of sexual activity and recreational drug use. Some donate blood to be stored for their own use later.

Behind the Call for Screening

Because there is no known cure for AIDS, most efforts today aim at reducing the number of cases through prevention of transmission. Thus, debate over identifying HIV carriers has been sparked. Because many individuals infected with HIV experience no medical problems despite the presence of the virus, they are most likely to unwittingly transmit it to others through sexual activity or sharing needles. Fear of transmission throughout much of the population has led many to call for screening to identify people who are seropositive for HIV and who therefore could transmit the virus to others.

That a certain amount of screening for HIV and AIDS should be done elicits little argument. When specifics are discussed, however, emotionally charged differences arise over who should be tested, whether screening should be voluntary or mandatory, and how the test results should be used.

Why Screen?

Screening is done for many reasons. As a medical tool, it is used (1) to help understand what is wrong with a patient, (2) to make an accurate diagnosis, (3) to provide information that helps in reaching a particular decision, (4) to ensure compliance and control after a problem has been treated, (5) to promote public safety, or (6) to gather research for scientific purposes.

For diagnostic purposes, screening may help identify a particular disease or problem. One criterion for diagnosing an AIDS patient is to screen for the presence of HIV antibodies. In part, this helps to confirm the diagnosis of AIDS even when other medical problems are evident. In this way, screening for HIV antibodies in a patient suspected of having AIDS is not much different from screening for other medical problems.

Screening also may help provide necessary medical information. A clear and legitimate use of screening techniques for individuals is found in the field of genetics, where people are screened to determine whether or not they carry defective genes that could affect their children. The resulting information can help people reach procreative decisions different from those decisions they might make without the knowledge afforded by the test.

Similar screening has been suggested for people at high or low risk for HIV. Through screening, intravenous drug abusers, people who have had blood transfusions since 1977, and homosexuals or bisexuals may obtain information that could affect their sexual practices, procreative decisions, and behaviors that place others at risk for infection.

A common reason to screen in both medical and nonmedical settings is to monitor the behavior of a person in whom society places its trust. The medical professional discovered to be abusing alcohol or other drugs, for example, may be required to go through a rehabilitation program. After completing the program, professionals may be screened at random intervals to check for the presence of controlled substances or alcohol in their bodies. The purpose is to protect patients from harm that may be caused by impairment of a person responsible for their medical treatment. Other professionals are screened because of the value of their work and the potential danger to and vulnerability of an unsuspecting public. Society decides that protection of the patient or the public is vital.

In promoting public safety, screening also is used to protect the integrity of the nation's blood supply. Once AIDS was recognized as a threat and a useful method of screening for HIV was developed, all donated blood became subject to the screening.

In addition, screening may be part of an epidemiological study to help health officials and others in public life promote the safety and well-being of society and inhibit the spread of disease. When cures or other avenues of care are available, it is easier to justify this kind of screening. Yet, even with random HIV screening, society may benefit from better information about how many people are HIV positive and how many may become ARC and AIDS patients. It may provide a way to project and plan for the cost of their healthcare and perhaps even help researchers more clearly understand the exact paths of transmission, factors that contribute to the disease, and therapies or drugs that may be useful in treating HIV, ARC, and AIDS.

Screening, then, can be useful and beneficial. When the information it provides is abused, however, screening also can be harmful and destructive. The act of screening is the simplest part of the equation. Managing the resulting information and caring for people is more difficult. The most ethically responsible decisions can be reached only by seriously weighing the alternatives. Ethics committees are one forum for healthcare institutions to address the issues.

Broad-Based vs. Targeted Groups

Those who support broad-based screening argue that because the AIDS virus is transmitted sexually (through a strong human drive) or through blood and blood products (essential to every life) identifying individuals who could transmit the virus is important. With knowledge of their HIV seropositivity, proponents argue, carriers probably will change their behavior or could be isolated in an effort to avoid transmitting the virus.

The key question, opponents argue, is whether or not information alone is sufficient to motivate people to change sexual practices, intravenous drug abuse, and other actions that place others at risk. There are already current examples of known HIV carriers who chose not to notify later sexual partners that the contact placed them at risk. Also, fear of isolation could drive those at greatest risk underground to avoid tests and live in ignorance of their condition.

Those who argue against wide screening also point out the enormous financial costs and that, at best, a negative test confirms that on the day of the screening, a person was not HIV positive. The HIV test cannot predict which individuals will convert to a seropositive condition in a short time. A clean bill of health today cannot guarantee that a person's actions tomorrow will not expose him or her to the virus. Also, if exposure to HIV occurred shortly before the test, the virus will not necessarily show up on the day of the test. Medical science is not sure whether a person can transmit the virus during the time between exposure to HIV and conversion to seropositivity.

Some people favor selective screening of groups considered most at risk of contracting HIV. Others are suspicious about how individuals in those groups would be identified and treated, particularly because today's high-risk patients in the United States fall into categories that generally are not socially acceptable. Given that homosexuals, bisexuals, and intravenous drug abusers as "classes" of people are generally pushed to the outskirts of social life and often hide their orientation, how could these persons be made to undergo HIV testing? And to what forms of discrimination would even noninfected members be subjected?

In any case, designations of groups as high or low risk will blur rapidly when HIV spreads among heterosexuals. Although it is still true that only a small percentage of all HIV-seropositive patients contracted the virus through heterosexual activity, their numbers are increasing. In many other areas of the world, transmission of the virus has been primarily through heterosexual activity. What happens when these people visit the United States or try to immigrate here? Should HIV-seropositive individuals be denied admission to the United States?

Further, since death becomes imminent for any AIDS patient, should every patient be tested on admission to any healthcare institution so that healthcare workers can be advised to take proper precautions? For that matter, should every healthcare worker be tested so that co-workers and patients are protected? Should seropositivity be sufficient grounds to dismiss or reassign certain categories of healthcare professionals, for example, those with direct patient contact?

Voluntary vs. Mandatory

Once agreement is reached on who should be tested, the argument turns to whether the screening should be voluntary or mandatory. Ethics committees discussing AIDS screening should be guided by similar questions attendant to other situations, such as worker safety, employee physical examinations, and high-risk factors.

Each argument already has precedent in public policy. To keep the U.S. blood supply as clean as possible, every blood donation is mandatorily screened. Generally, voluntary screening is encouraged for people in high-risk groups. The U.S. military has mandated HIV screening for all applicants to the services based on the possibility that enlistees may be called on to donate blood in a time of crisis or war, and that contaminated blood would only compromise the nation's chances for survival.

Some argue that every healthcare worker and every patient should undergo mandatory testing to protect others from inadvertently contracting the AIDS virus. Mandatory testing, then, can be prescribed for specific classes of individuals, such as those who are at high or low risk, or it can be done for specific reasons, such as the desire to keep HIV out of the blood supply. The ethical underpinning of the argument is that the innocent are protected, whereas those who need help are identified.

Another argument for mandatory testing revolves around the seriousness of AIDS and the nature of the disease. Because no cure exists and because people who contract full-blown AIDS die, society must be protected from AIDS as from other infectious or sexually transmitted diseases. This argument is the base on which mandatory testing is suggested for certain groups of people, such as all hospital patients or all people who apply for marriage licenses. Ethical values of society, life, and family are voiced. Many who have daily contact with hospital patients contend that knowledge of whether a particular patient carries HIV or suffers from ARC or AIDS is vital to both the proper care of the patient and the protection of the healthcare worker. Similarly, the argument goes, people about to marry have the right to enter the new relationship knowing whether or not they are at risk, and they have the duty not to produce children who may be born with the virus.

When Results Test Positive: Patients' Rights vs. Public Health

As complicated as the AIDS epidemic is, healthcare professionals must help balance the rights of each patient against the general good of the public. If HIV test results are inaccurate, what impact will they have on individuals, families, and society as a whole? Conversely, what impact will accurate results engender? How will society deal with the occasional incident of HIV transmission after testing shows negative?

Must the person who tests seropositive be given the information? If so, who should tell the person, and where should the results be sent? Should others, such as current and former sexual partners, be told? What should be done for the seropositive person? Little can be done for sufferers of AIDS or ARC. If the person only carries the HIV virus, however, there is no certainty that he or she will either become fatally ill or stay well. In seeking to stop transmission of the virus, should society determine whether the seropositive person must abstain from sex altogether, or whether "safer sex" can be practiced? Can such determinations be reasonably monitored, let alone enforced?

Ethical Questions to Ask

In addressing the ethical issues, it is important to define (1) what any screening is to be used for, (2) why it is to be used, (3) in what specific way the resulting information will be used, (4) and how the values of the person being screened can be protected. For example, in promoting public health and safety, how far can, or should, the state carry its obligation to protect the health and welfare of its citizens in general? Should that obligation override individual freedom, privacy, or rights of patients to conquer contagious diseases?

Based on the premise of promoting public safety, should HIV carriers be isolated from the rest of the population or even identified at all on a large scale? It is difficult to justify screening an entire population for HIV seropositivity when presence of the virus does not necessarily indicate sickness. Will mass screening for HIV really promote public health, or will the results merely provide information that will be used for discriminatory purposes? Or will the information both promote public health and provide discrimination? If both occur, do the benefits of one outweigh the drawbacks of the other?

Informed Consent

Other ethical issues must be considered, especially informed consent. Must a person be notified and agree in advance that he or she will be tested for HIV? If so, how must consent be obtained?

Some people argue that specific informed consent is not necessary for the HIV test. They argue that a person who signs a general consent form when entering a hospital, for instance, does not need to sign an additional sheet specifically stating that the HIV test can be done. The Red Cross procedure of routinely testing blood and blood products for HIV antibodies supports this argument, since specific informed consent is not required of the donor. The fact that blood is volunteered presumes consent.

On the other hand, others argue that because of the nature and severity of AIDS and the possible consequences of a positive result, individuals should know about and approve of any testing in advance. Generally, this group thinks that the physician should discuss the test and that the patient should sign a form before any HIV testing is done.

Where and by Whom?

Another ethical issue involves where and by whom HIV testing is done. Currently, many people are tested either by the Red Cross when they donate blood or at hospitals when they check in as patients. However, serious questions arise about whether testing also should be provided elsewhere, such as at clinics for sexually transmitted diseases, or physicians' office buildings, or public health clinics. Whose responsibility is it to provide information about test results? Who should be notified? The more mandatory the screening, the more public facilities will be required to provide such services. As hospitals diversify their activities and acquire or manage nonacute care programs, these issues arise.

Who Pays? Who Gets Results?

Still another issue is expense. Who should pay for HIV testing? If it is the taxpayers as a whole or patients individually, are the financial resources available? If screening is being done only for private information so a person knows whether or not the disease may be transmitted, should the public have to pay the bill? If a critically ill patient enters a hospital and is found to have AIDS or ARC, should the test be considered similar to any other diagnostic test and be reimbursed by an insurance company? And if an insurance company pays for the testing, does it have the right to know the test results and perhaps change insurance coverage, increase premiums, or cancel policies altogether?

The issue of cost, therefore, raises another ethical issue: confidentiality of test results. Once results have been determined, who should get them? Should it be only the physician? Should results be sent through the laboratory of a hospital? Confidentiality is meant to ensure the trusting relationship between physician and patient so that healthcare needs may best be met. Any compromise of confidentiality between patient and physician, or between patient and any healthcare provider, seriously undermines the ability to deliver quality care.

HIV-positive patients' rights still must be weighed against the need for a safe healthcare environment for both non-HIV patients and providers. Patients should have the right to confidentiality, autonomy, and access to healthcare regardless of the nature of their illness. Healthcare workers and non-HIV patients should have the right to protect themselves against infection through accident, dirty needles, or contact with the bodily fluids of AIDS, ARC, and HIV-positive patients. More than in other areas, a person's HIV seropositivity raises delicate questions of balancing an individual's civil liberties against the values and rights of employees, the requirements of a safe workplace, and public health.

Charting Seropositivity

A key question arises over whether or not positive HIV test results should be placed on a patient's chart, especially if the patient does not suffer from AIDS or ARC. Should positive results be part of the chart so that individuals who treat or care for the patient can take appropriate precautions to protect themselves? Or, to protect the patient's confidentiality, should the chart read only that healthcare personnel should follow blood and body fluid precautions appropriate to infection control? Should the specific results be included on the chart as a valuable piece of information that may give clues to later diagnostic work by a physician or paraprofessional? Or, since HIV-positive status is not in itself a disease, and the patient may be hospitalized for some other condition, should a positive result be left off the chart?

Finally, some argue that because charted evidence of a positive test result probably would trigger a potentially catastrophic loss of the patient's insurance, the medical ethics of the situation call for the information to be shielded or protected. Others argue that it is not the place of medical professionals to make those decisions, but rather to care for the patient regardless of insurability.

How Far to Follow Up?

The issue of confidentiality and charting positive test results has to distinguish between the HIV-positive person and the patient suffering from ARC or AIDS. People suffering from ARC or AIDS are, by definition, seropositive to HIV. This information is vital to both the medical treatment of the patient and the safety of healthcare workers.

Other variations on confidentiality become even more striking when questions arise as to whether or not seropositive results should be shared with a spouse, other sexual partners, intravenous drug users with whom an infected person may have shared needles, or someone who was in contact with the virus through a blood transfusion or other exposure to blood products. Does society have a right, as it does with other sexually transmitted diseases, to follow up on and notify an infected individual's sexual contacts that a partner has been confirmed as positive for HIV?

Research

A final area of ethical concern involves research. A major problem with AIDS is that so much about it is unknown, particularly about why some HIV-positive people contract ARC or AIDS and others do not. Much data must be gathered to help understand such mysteries as the spread of the virus throughout society, the nature of risk groups, and the method of transmission from female to male. As with all research involving human subjects, specific informed consent must be obtained and forms signed voluntarily by the infected person or his or her proxy. Failure to do so compromises the research subject and would represent a bold and unethical step beyond the accepted bounds of human research.

Conclusion

AIDS threatens a segment of society with death. Stopping the transmission of the deadly virus is an important item on the U.S. health agenda. Screening represents one discussion of how to accomplish this goal.

Screening has limits. Defining the goals and projecting the values of any anticipated action are critical factors that should be clarified before any screening program is implemented. The danger is that emotion will overpower reason. When life is threatened, emotional reaction is natural, but the need for reasoned discussion becomes even greater.

As in any other discussion of ethical issues, it is difficult to recognize and consider all values, but that is must be done. Articulating the reasons to pursue certain values over others will help establish the scope, direction, and quality of any screening program, especially one involving HIV.

AZT and AIDS 24

Research protocols on AZT, a drug that holds some promise for treatment of AIDS patients, were halted even as the federal Food and Drug Administration (FDA) gave permission for the drug to be prescribed for AIDS sufferers. Quick FDA approval of a promising but not thoroughly tested drug offers some hope to patients who previously had none. Termination of the drug trials, however, raises more serious questions of medical ethics:

- How can the true efficacy of a drug such as AZT be discovered without study of its long-term effects?
- How can valid questions about the drug's adverse effects or intrinsic value be addressed?
- At what cost was the clinical trial stopped?
- Should perceived benefits for some take precedence over thorough testing that expands knowledge, detects limitations, and traces potential long-term side effects?
- Should all AIDS patients be guaranteed access to AZT, now that it has been FDA approved? If so, who should bear the expense?

The drug trials were halted because some human research subjects experienced benefits while taking AZT. The significance of these benefits, whether merely perceived or real, was heightened by the reality that there is currently neither a cure for AIDS nor any other FDA-approved drug available to manage the disease. In addition, because so many AIDS patients are young and AZT offers the potential to prolong their lives, any attendant risk seems worthwhile. Consequently, standard concerns accompanying drug testing and clinical experimentation were set aside in favor of patient benefit.

Ethicists question how to strike a balance between the continued need for sound scientific study of AZT treatment against the needs of extremely ill individuals who require immediate therapy. When only one approved drug offers hope at this time, who has the right to deny it to patients who surely will die without it? By the same token, who has the right to stop experimentation with other experimental drugs whose effects are still unknown?

Problems Hit Home

Many healthcare institutions will face medical, ethical, and financial quandaries about continued AZT therapy. This involves patients who were taking the drug at no cost through a research protocol and who wish to continue the therapy. These patients cannot afford AZT, however, now that the drug has been approved by the FDA. As institutions grapple with how to handle the medical and financial aspects of AIDS and AZT, they also must consider the ethical issues of continued treatment.

Justice should be a major concern with AZT administration. Should an institution or clinic cease to provide the drug because of cost? Should it provide AZT to all patients who need it, regardless of their ability to pay, even if it means using resources also needed elsewhere? And since AZT is expensive, should an institution be prepared to provide the drug to all, even if it endangers the institution's viability?

AZT undoubtedly will be the first of many drugs that eventually will be developed to treat AIDS patients. When other drugs are available, probably also at high cost, how will decisions be made to pay for some or all patients? And will people suffering from cancer, heart disease, or other life-threatening illnesses be given the same consideration?

Research

Research on human beings often is necessary to advance medical care and to help patients. AIDS is a case in point. History shows that many beneficial vaccines and other therapies, such as smallpox and poliomyelitis vaccines, open heart surgery, and successful treatment of birth defects, have resulted only after research on humans beings.

Compelling evidence shows, however, that human research has been abused at times in various countries, including the United States. In particular, abuses associated with Nazi Germany in World War II serve as grim reminders of the necessity for good research protocols, ethical standards, and the need for monitoring.

To Heal or to Learn?

Research on human subjects is of two types, therapeutic and nontherapeutic. The primary purpose of nontherapeutic research is not to heal, but to learn. This is a significant problem when evaluating AZT experimentation and poses the following questions:

- What was being accomplished with AZT research treatments before the FDA put the drug on the approved list?
- Was this therapy for human subjects, or was it to learn about the possible efficacy of AZT in AIDS patients?
- Was AZT experimentation done to learn more about how the drug interacts with the virus and how it affects people?
- When no other therapy is available, can one automatically assume that the experiment is therapeutic, that is, a study to measure the drug's efficacy and to promote healing?
- Was AZT used purely for research, or did it have a significant therapeutic benefit?
- Did the perceived benefit of AZT as a therapy for AIDS patients seem greater because it was the only drug that offered hope in treating this fatal disease?

Some research can be therapeutic. There is a strong argument that AZT treatment was a therapeutic research protocol and that both types of research could have been involved since no cure was forthcoming. With AZT, the search was for knowledge about a drug's potential effect on AIDS in people manifesting certain clinical symptoms; therefore, the research was nontherapeutic. At the same time, many hoped for therapeutic benefit that would improve AIDS patients' health and delay their death. In such situations, according to this argument, one may assume greater risks if the research is directed toward healing as well as knowledge. Thus, with therapeutic AZT research, great risks could be undertaken despite toxicity or other long-range complications that might not be acceptable for a nontherapeutic drug trial.

Despite this compelling argument, the dissenting group offers the following questions:

- Is AZT or any other future drug for AIDS really beneficial?

- If so, is the benefit measured in hope or in proven effective treatment?
- What are the differences between the short-term and long-term results of this drug use?
- Are there side effects that will be unacceptably harmful to patients if they begin to take the drug too early?
- Will the drug's toxicity lessen the quality of an individual's life if the patient must take it for a prolonged time?

Underlying all these questions is a major concern: they cannot be answered until the research protocol has been completed.

Maintaining Principles

In evaluating the ethical norms involved in trying to reach some conclusions about the ethical acceptability of research on human beings, the following principles may be helpful.

1. The knowledge sought must be important and not obtainable by any other means. Also the research must be conducted by qualified people. In the case of AZT or other drugs proposed for use by AIDS patients or others suffering from life-threatening illness, these key questions must be answered appropriately: Have all laboratory studies been completed? Have the necessary studies on animals and/or cadavers been completed? Is there sufficient reason to believe that the drug holds real promise of efficacy in treating the disease? Is there any way other than experimenting on human beings to discover this information? Unless these questions are answered truthfully and positively, drug trials on human beings should not be conducted.

2. The risk of suffering or injury to the subject must be proportionate to the benefit that may be gained. This principle becomes particularly important in examining the ethical nature of nontherapeutic experimentation with human beings. Can the harm of agreeing to a research protocol be justified when no benefit is to be gained for the human subject? In the case of AZT and other treatments that promise some hope, the risk of suffering or injury becomes more acceptable because of the

potential benefits to the human research subjects. In addition, when a disease is uniformly fatal, individuals may be willing to accept huge risk and great possibility of suffering or pain in exchange for the hope of finding a cure, gaining some relief, or prolonging life.

3. The research subjects must be selected so that the risks and benefits will not fall unequally on one group in society. This does not appear to have been a problem in the case of AZT research. Most individuals with full-blown AIDS who may have been able to benefit from the treatment, given the opportunity to enter the research protocol, would not have been selected disproportionately from among minorities or the poor. However, a related problem arises once the research protocol has been completed or stopped and the drug approved by the FDA. In some states, AZT is not covered by government-sponsored insurance programs, raising the danger that only those who can pay for it will be able to obtain the drug. In the interest of justice, can a drug be withheld from needy patients who have inadequate financial resources to pay for it?

Further, what about those indigent patients who participated in the first phase of AZT drug trials? Should they be given greatest or least priority for obtaining the drug now that it is on the market? Should every effort be made to continue the drug, even if they cannot pay for it, because they may already have experienced some benefit? Or should other poor patients who have not had the opportunity to participate in the research now be targeted for the FDA-approved drug? Should there be a commitment to treating all AIDS sufferers who request AZT, regardless of financial consequences? Many hospitals treating AIDS patients have confronted this issue already, since some states do not cover AZT under Medicaid programs. In addition, the waiting period sometimes is so long that the patient dies before the drug can be used. These issues of discrimination must be addressed carefully.

4. Issues of informed consent must be respected. In experimentation, complications surrounding informed consent arise because of the nature of research. Research requires compari-

son; some patients may be given a placebo. In double-blind studies, even the researcher does not know which therapy is administered and what benefit, if any, the therapy may have. The purpose of the research would be defeated if the patient knew the true treatment category. Nevertheless, any potential subject of experimentation should be informed as fully as possible about what to expect, what perceived benefits and risks may accrue, and what is not known about a drug such as AZT.

Similar guidelines cover proxy consent, with an important exception. A person with the power of proxy consent should never permit, or be permitted to agree to, nontherapeutic treatment that uses an individual simply because the patient is incompetent or otherwise incapable of speaking for himself or herself.

5. A human research subject must be free to terminate involvement in experimental treatment protocols at any time. This ensures that informed consent is respected and that people are not treated unfairly or against their will.

6. There must be a commitment to seek good, accurate results, with research brought to an appropriate conclusion. This is the primary issue raised with the termination of AZT clinical trials. Was the information gleaned in the short trial time adequate to draw sound scientific and medical conclusions about the efficacy of AZT? A negative answer makes it difficult to justify termination of the research, even with the hope of benefits available to seriously ill individuals.

If the AZT precedent is followed as other AIDS-related drugs are developed, marketed, and tested, the problem will be magnified. When four or five different drugs are on the market, with each offering some benefit but none conclusively tested, what new problems will be raised; not only in terms of unknown side effects, but what problems in terms of access, economics, and justice within individual hospitals and clinics?

Future AIDS Research

Much attention has focused on AIDS and AIDS-related research seeking both to learn more about the virus and to discover potentially beneficial medical interventions. Initially, AZT was a promising drug for a group of people who suffer from AIDS. However, the hopeful start and the attendant pressure to take the drug out of experimental status may raise more complicated problems in the long run. Answers to questions about toxicity, efficacy, and long-term results may not be answered properly because of the short-circuited clinical trial.

In evaluating drug trials for AIDS patients, one of the most difficult issues facing ethics committees is how to weigh the benefits and risks of treatment of such a devastating disease. Is it true that, if one is going to die anyway from a disease with no known cure, any step that carries some promise or hope is worth the risk? When confronted with a communicable, life-threatening illness, is it ethically possible to deny some people a certain drug because noninfected "experts" believe it has not been tested thoroughly enough? Is it realistic or legitimate to propose accurate scientific information and solid medical knowledge as a value that should override a patient's desperate desire for a drug that offers hope?

Conclusion

There is one fundamental commandment in healthcare ethics: treat all individuals with compassion, care, hope, respect, and dignity. This applies especially to patients who are imminently dying. Treating people with compassion, however, must not be confused with jumping to conclusions, embracing inconclusive data, or conveying false hope. It is difficult enough to help people deal with a devastating and fatal disease without having to manage the bitterness that inevitably accompanies the shattering of false promises.

AZT raises the first of many questions that will be asked as new protocols are developed for treating AIDS, ARC, and HIV seropositive patients. The brunt of the ethical questions will fall on the professionals who care for these patients both in and out of the healthcare institution. Ultimate decisions about what drugs or treatments to offer will rest with attending physicians and with financial officers responsible for allocating available healthcare dollars. Ethics committees can help now, however, by focusing discussion and raising awareness of the serious issues that must be addressed before decisions can be made.

Organan Transplants: Small   25
Supply vs. Great Demand

To the public, it was a great breakthrough, a demonstration of technological and medical skill that fostered visions of immortality. To the medical community, Dr. David Hume's first series of kidney transplants in the early 1950s brought ethical and political questions along with the dynamic new surgical procedure. How great would be society's commitment to continue organ transplants? How great would be its commitment to finance transplants? Where would donors be found? At what point could an organ be taken from one person and given to another? How full a life would transplant recipients be able to live?

Representatives of all healthcare institutions, both large and small, must consider the ethical issues that arise in this expanding area of organ transplants. The promise of life and the scarcity of organs require all health providers to deal with the issues surrounding organ transplantation.[1]

Live Donors: How Informed Their Consent?

One of a live donor's paired organs offers the greatest benefit to the recipient because the rejection factor can be minimized if the donor is a good match. Organ transplants that occur between identical twins are the most successful. After identical twins, histologically compatible relatives are the best donors; as with twins, they reduce the rejection factor and offer the recipient the greatest chance for a rewarding quality of life. But, how does a potential donor decide whether to donate a kidney?

Informed consent is the greatest ethical issue that arises in the donation of a paired organ. Informed consent means that an individual is told of both risks and benefits that can arise in a particular procedure. Because relatives offer the best histological compatibility, tremendous pressure is placed on a potential donor. This can have an impact on the ability to obtain informed consent.

Risks to the donor are difficult to list. Individuals must be cautioned about the possibility of unforeseen, adverse events. For example, the donor may be willing to give up one kidney for the life of a relative. The donor, however, would then have no backup in case of later injury or disease involving the remaining kidney. If an adverse event were to occur, the donor may resent having given consent; family relationships could suffer. Even without such an event, a sense of obligation for the gift of an organ could substantially alter the relationship between recipient and donor. A refusal can fracture an entire family.

Assent, however, creates additional considerations for healthcare institutions and physicians. With more than one patient involved, which one's needs take priority, the donor's or the recipient's?

Informed consent must be obtained despite these obstacles. Attention to the primary patient, whether recipient or donor, is essential. Institutional ethics committees must address these issues.

Cadaver Organs: Limited Resource

Organs from a dead person pose different ethical problems, the first being determination of death. In the United States, brain death is a valid criterion. This requires death of the entire brain, that is, both neocortical and brainstem functions. In a small percentage of patients, this will occur while artificial life-support systems continue cardiopulmonary functions—a necessary procedure to maintain organs in the best possible condition. Medical care of the dead patient must be maintained until the harvest team arrives to take the organs and transport them to the transplant center.

Some people fear signing organ-transplant cards because they think their care near death will be only minimal or substandard so their organs can be taken sooner. Institutions must ensure that (1) care is never compromised while a person is dying, (2) that the donor is never used to promote the life of the recipient in an unethical manner, and (3) appropriate education is offered to the community.

The primary issue in cadaver donation, as with live donors, is informed consent. Since 1968, the United States has operated under The Uniform Anatomical Gift Act, which allows individuals to donate specific organs or their whole body for use in organ transplants or medical science. The act is based on a notion of charity: individuals, in their goodness, desire to bequeath their organs to others. Institutions may find that even though individuals may have signed organ donation statements, family members may deny the request. Each institution must develop methods to secure the gift of organs.

A less frequently raised ethical issue lies in the measure of obligation placed on individuals in case of traumatic death. Is the donation of organs simply a matter of charity? Does a special moral obligation rest on every person? Can the emotional needs of a family overturn another's sense of obligation to donate organs? The problem can be resolved if each institution develops a way to ask the family what the dying person might have wanted rather than what the family wants.

Informed consent can be coerced in two ways: either for or against organ donation. The donor can be coerced into giving organs on the basis of charity or the law, or the donor can be coerced into not giving organs based on fear of poor care near the time of death. Both are unethical.

New Way of Life for Recipients

Organ recipients also confront the issue of informed consent. Their most difficult task is understanding the life changes that receiving a transplant will entail. Unlike other medical procedures, transplantation is not a question of undergoing a particular surgical procedure, leaving the hospital, and living with a quality of life similar to that before surgery. The recipient must understand the issues of continued drug therapy, dependence on technology, shortened life span, and other psychological, social, and familial concerns.

Informed consent as total understanding is impossible for the organ recipient. However, every institution that performs organ transplants must establish an educational process to promote reasonable understanding by recipients. This must include information on the quality and type of life after a successful transplant, the effect it will have on other dimensions of life, and an understanding of the years available after the transplant.

Who Receives Organs?

Given the scarcity of organs and the large number of people awaiting them, a just system of distribution must be established. Logically, only those who will benefit medically from a transplant should receive one. This requires the elimination of intractable smokers (for heart transplants) or severe alcoholics (for liver transplants). In these situations environmental or lifestyle issues prevent the recipient from benefiting from a scarce resource. Use of a limited number of organs for these individuals when others can benefit does not make sense.

Another issue is that of therapy vs. experimentation. Presently, some organ transplants, such as corneas, kidneys, and hearts, are therapeutic. Others, such as livers, pancreas, and lungs, are still experimental. Experimental procedures have larger unanswered questions, including appropriate rehabilitative long term care, quality of life, expected longevity, pharmacologic needs, and psychological problems.

The ability to comply with appropriate follow-up care is another issue. Those who lack support in their personal lives, or those who indicate that they are not willing to comply with a strict medical regimen after transplant, may be refused a transplant. It is the transplant team's decision to determine the limits of necessary medical compliance. This criterion could easily be abused; understanding social factors is not easy. In those situations where clear and ample evidence shows compliance will not occur, however, it is unjust to waste a scarce resource.

The distribution of organs must be just. Public relations and media hype should not be the basis for distribution. In 1986, much was made of Baby Jesse's need for a heart in Loma Linda, CA. Although front pages of newspapers and nightly national news broadcasts gave much coverage of this case, there were other children, including Baby Calvin in Louisville, KY, who had been on waiting lists longer. Nonetheless, the media hype over Baby Jesse provided him with a heart before Baby Calvin received one, even though Baby Calvin had been on a waiting list at a referral center before Baby Jesse was born. The same can be said of using political clout.

Who receives transplants is also a question of money. It is important for society to examine whether the wealthy's ability to pay represents an undesirable advantage in obtaining transplants. The question of wealthy people from outside the United States receiving scarce organs highlights this issue more vividly.

Public Policy and Organ Donation

With the active involvement of the healthcare community, U.S. public policy needs to address some of these issues.

1. *Allocating a scarce resource.* This involves asking questions about distributive justice. Who receives organ transplants? How can distribution be made equitable so that rich and poor, black and white, young and old, and men and women receive transplants? What ensures that wealth and power are not the criteria for allocating an organ? Healthcare institutions that resolve these issues can give needed direction to the national debate.

Determinations based on social worth or social criteria must be avoided. It is nothing more than guesswork to say that one person is worth more than another because of past experience or future promise. Criteria that emphasize reasoned choices need to be established to help eliminate feelings of rejection or worthlessness on the part of those not chosen. Justice can prevail only if choices are made on the basis of medical benefit, need, and fairness.

2. *Financing research.* How much money should be allocated for study in the face of other healthcare needs in the United States? In an open system of healthcare financing, it is difficult to make tradeoffs. Institutional decisions will determine where money will be spent. Should primary and secondary care take precedence over continued technological advances? Public poli-

cy needs to address the priorities that healthcare spending will take. In general, focus on primary care and wellness will serve the nation's health more than will these technologies. Balancing these choices is on the agenda for public debate.

3. *Deciding who should pay?* Financing healthcare is a thorny issue. In the early 1970s, the United States decided to finance hemodialysis and kidney transplants. Consequently, no one in need is denied financial assistance for these procedures. The present discussion surrounding financing liver and heart transplants reflects the inadequacy of that solution.

Public policy responds to the values society wishes to pursue. But should public funds be used to finance organ transplant experimentation when the government has no intention of financing the successful result of the research? If society continues to foster the development of this technology, it must be willing to provide access for all. This can take the form of public money or facilitating financing at local levels through funds, centers, and regulations.

Another financial issue is the selling of organs. This suggestion has been made to alleviate the shortage of organs. From an ethical perspective, however, the notion of selling organs is unfair. Wealthy people would not be tempted to sell their organs, whereas those under financial hardship may be too willing to place their lives on the line.

4. *Chooosing where to transplant.* A final policy concern is where organ transplants take place. Growing numbers of transplant services within institutions may be counterproductive. Transplant centers with reliable statistics, sound experimental protocols, and experienced providers may offer the finest results. Societal structures will have to be developed to provide equal access to those transplant centers that provide the highest quality of care and greatest use of a scarce resource.

What Healthcare Centers Can Do

Institutions should participate in procuring organs for transplants. In every healthcare institution, patients who could be valuable donors die. Each institution must establish a protocol for requesting organs. The size of an institution does not excuse it from these concerns.

Also, individual hospitals may stimulate community support and discussion. Education about the need for organs has not been thorough or successful. Community discussions led by hospitals can help ensure that excellent care will be given to the dying while organs are harvested for others.

Conclusion

Unless ethics committees grapple with these issues as an overall policy in the educational structure of their institutions, social debate will not take place. More importantly, the increasing opportunity to provide extended life for human beings will be lost.

1. Dale Cowan et al., *Human Organ Transplantation: Societal, Medical-Legal, Regulatory, and Reimbursement Issues,* Health Administration Press, Ann Arbor, MI, 1987.

Does One Have a Right to Stop Artificial Nutrition and Hydration?

26

Is it ever permissible to withdraw or withhold food and liquid from a person? Is food a medical therapy or a human necessity? Is it murder to withhold or withdraw food, knowing that certain death will follow? Is it suicide to request that food and water not be used at some point in the future? Every acute and long term healthcare institution faces these issues. Each institution must weigh the arguments of all positions.

Arguments for Requiring Nutrition and Hydration

The argument that nutrition and hydration must be provided to every person, regardless of extenuating circumstances, is usually framed in one or more of the following ways. The first is that nutrition and hydration are normal aspects of human care. Basic "nursing care" or "medical care" require that a patient or resident be provided with some nutrition and hydration; otherwise, this argument concludes, the person is starved to death. This is unethical.

Some people argue that withdrawing or withholding nutrition and hydration, unlike other medical therapies, leads to certain death. In removing a ventilator, for example, a person may continue to breathe. In removing a feeding therapy, however, a person will surely die. To deny nutrition or hydration, therefore, is to hasten death. This argument equates withdrawing or withholding nutrition to a form of euthanasia, which is a denial of the ethical tenets of medicine as a profession. Another position states that situations may arise when forced feeding or hydration is not ethically required. But such decisions will start society on a "slippery slope," which will result in the "death by starvation" of all unwanted citizens because they are impaired, useless, too burdensome to care for, or require too much of society's economic resources.[1] The wholesale death of the weak and infirm must not be allowed. Therefore, this argument concludes, no person can be allowed to forego nutrition or hydration.

Some would argue that because eating is a social activity during which family, friendship, love, and human values are celebrated and shared, this symbol could be lost or denied. The symbolic and emotional sensitivities to life, according to this stance, should make us question whether one can allow a person to die by withdrawing or denying normal nutrition and hydration.

Closely associated with these concerns is the position that dehydration and starvation are painful, agonizing, and inhumane. The ugliness of death under these circumstances argues against the denial of food and water. Some also argue that there is great pain for the patient in these situations, although this is not always true.

Some people place the continued promotion of the value of life as a greater value for the common good. Allowing the withholding or withdrawal of nutrition and hydration places society's promotion of human life in jeopardy. Denying a patient or surrogate the right to refuse nutrition and hydration is one way of supporting the value and dignity of each person's life.

Finally, some argue that because the law is so uncertain in this area, patients must be hydrated and fed by any means until there is some consensus on the issue in the legal community. The difficulty with this argument is that it rests on a false premise, that ethical and medical practices are secondary to the law or that ethical and medical conflicts can be resolved by the law. The law has its appropriate place, but it is not necessarily the best "final arbitrator."

With the exception of the final argument, each of these arguments has some merit. Each expresses basic values important to medicine as a profession, to society, or to patients and their families. The questions each institution must ask in dealing with these problems concern the validity and truthfulness of the assumptions made in the arguments.

Arguments for Withholding and Withdrawing

The argument that nutrition and hydration can be denied in certain circumstances is based on a concept with a different group of statements. One set of arguments equates nutrition and hydration therapy to the curative process. This argument states that since useless treatments are not appropriate, nutrition and hydration may be withdrawn or withheld. If there is an underlying condition that cannot be cured (e.g., the collapse of the digestive system), the provision of nutrition and hydration will not cure the primary problem. In addition, the secondary problems are such that all one can achieve through nutrition and hydration is to prolong the physical functions of life with no hope of cure.

An associated argument centers on prolonging the dying process. The irreversibly comatose patient may be force-fed, but what occurs over the months or years is not the curative or caring goals of medicine, but rather the prolonging of the patient's death. When it is medically determined that the person's comatose state is irreversible, nutrition and hydration take on different meaning. They are no longer being used to provide nutrition while the person's other diseases are being healed.

Another argument relates to the wishes of the patient and the burdens of the treatment. In some cases, patients or residents make it clear that they do not wish to be force-fed at the end of their lives. Some even make valiant efforts to remove feeding tubes, whether nasogastric tubes or surgically implanted gastrostomy tubes. The person perceives the feeding mechanism as too burdensome. Burdens include pain, loss of mobility, decreased quality of life, and economic concerns. In these circumstances, according to this argument, nutrition and hydration may be withheld or withdrawn.

The arguments for selective withholding or withdrawal of nutrition and hydration are based on several basic assumptions. First is the assumption that nutrition and hydration therapy is medical intervention, and that the decision to employ such treatment should be based on the same criteria as any other medical treatment. Additionally, a difference exists between fulfilling a stated or implied request for nutrition and hydration and imposing nutrition and hydration on the patient who requests to have such feedings withheld. Finally, the patient's total well-being is the primary medical concern.

Assumptions About Persons and Healthcare

To think about the issue from an ethical point of view, which may or may not be reflected in the law, one must address the assumptions made about the person, the profession of medicine, and healthcare.

Each person has various dimensions—physical, social, psychological, and spiritual. One must integrate all these dimensions to avoid dualistic and harmful ways of thinking. One aspect of the person is the physiological; the person's physical aspects must be seen as central since no person exists outside of a body. This concern is not necessarily the most important aspect of the person, since a person's body exists to help that person attain or pursue other values—spiritual, social, familial, and so on. As a result, maintaining the physical part of human life is an important value and responsibility, but not necessarily the ultimate value.

Care and responsibility for the human body include healthcare, nutrition, hydration, exercise, and cleanliness. One is not always able to do these things personally: infants and the senile and ill persons frequently require assistance. The family or society has a moral obligation to meet these needs. The ultimate goal in providing such care is to enable the person to realize human values to the greatest extent possible and not simply to maintain a physical body.

Medical care, including nutrition and hydration, would be offered to the ill person as part of the caring, curative, or comforting goals of the healthcare profession. The young child unable to feed herself or the older man needing assistance with sips of water would not be denied this because of lack of ability, strength, or usefulness. Appropriate care is a strong social and professional obligation.

A first conclusion about nutrition and hydration now can be made. One is not given or denied nutrition and hydration based on a personal ability to secure it for oneself. When a person, regardless of arbitrarily imposed standards such as intelligence, age, or productivity, is in need of food and water, there is a moral obligation to provide it.

Second, there are limits. Medicine, as a profession, pursues more than one goal. The most common goal is healing. Medical care seeks to restore a person to full, healthy life. A second goal is caring. A person suffering from chronic illness may be made comfortable which allows the pursuit of as many values in life as possible. Sometimes, however, neither goal is attainable. One can provide only comfort, relieving pain if it exists, and help the person to die with as much dignity as possible. Depending on which goal medical care is pursuing, therapies will be appropriate or inappropriate. For example, as the goal changes from healing to palliation, the appropriateness of a particular therapy can also change.

Central to the practice of medicine are the goals pursued with and for the patient. It is not the therapeutic intervention that captures our attention, but rather the needs and concerns of the person being treated. Thus, what is appropriate now may be inappropriate later. Nutrition and hydration therapies must be examined in the light of the patient's primary needs in the practice of medicine rather than as individual therapies. A time will come in each person's life when certain medical interventions are no longer necessary or appropriate.

Nutrition and Hydration Therapies

Nutrition and hydration therapies need to be evaluated in relation to the conceptions one has of medicine and of the person. The expressed needs of a patient for nutrition and hydration cannot be ignored on some arbitrary basis. One cannot starve a person to death when the word "starve" implies a deliberate and purposeful denial of nutrition and hydration to a person who cannot care for himself or herself. Implied in the obligation to feed and hydrate is a concern for more than the person's physical life. Healthcare is also concerned about the social, emotional, and creative dimensions of the patient.

Consistent with the comfort measures of medical care, nutrition and hydration should not be denied a person if these therapies provide pain relief. This requires a reexamination of expectations of normal intake, since small amounts of food and fluid may be all a person requires. As with other treatments, feeding therapies must be adjusted according to patient need. Thus, one can conclude, most patients should receive nutrition and hydration. For some patients, however, this is not valid. There is no moral obligation to continue or start treatments of any kind if the patient will be harmed or cannot benefit; the patient in a permanent vegetative state is one example. Maintaining the person in this manner focuses on the physical functions of the person alone, prolonging those functions when there is no hope for recovery of any other human functions. This can be considered useless therapy.

In circumstances when the patient will soon die, or the burdens associated with forced-feeding (as perceived by the patient) are great, there is no moral obligation to force-feed or hydrate. Latitude is needed in these situations because each person will decide differently. The focus of the decision, however, should be on the patient and the patient's needs, not on the therapy. As with other dying patients, cleanliness, pain relief (if any), and other basic care must be given.

Deciding Treatments

Those who argue that feeding and hydration must be given in all circumstances, despite the arguments just mentioned, have valid points for the healthcare protocols of many patients. Nonetheless, some choices must still be made. To argue that hydration and nutrition must be given because they are basic human care is to miss the significance of medically induced nutrition and hydration. The "slippery slope" argument or other symbolic elements in the decision to provide or withhold nutrition and hydration can lead to treatment inappropriate for the patient, although based on protection of the social good.

This claim is difficult to defend if one wishes to treat all people as an end and not as a means.

Finally, one cannot argue that because death will occur medical treatment cannot be withheld or withdrawn. The withdrawal or withholding of many treatments will result in death. The correct question is not whether death results, but whether one has an ethical obligation to prolong life by any means available.

Medical technology, including nutrition and hydration, requires careful decision making. Because medicine cannot always cure, each person eventually dies. Because illness is not the same for each person, different decisions must be made by society, the medical community, and patients.

From an ethical perspective, lines have to be drawn and different decisions made. To fail to make decisions about the withdrawal and withholding of nutrition and hydration is to avoid the issue. The difficult task facing each institution is to reach decisions regarding nutrition and hydration and to state clearly the reasons for those decisions.

---

1. William May et al., "Feeding and Hydrating the Permanently Unconscious and Other Vulnerable Persons," *Issues in Law and Medicine* 3:3, 1987, pp. 203–217.

Do-Not-Resuscitate Orders: 27
Revisited

Every person's heart stops eventually. This causes the cessation of all cardiopulmonary functions and is usually followed by a pronouncement of death. However, advances over the last 100 years enabled many individuals in and out of healthcare institutions to restart someone's heart after it stopped. The beginnings of cardiopulmonary resuscitation (CPR) are tied to the development of surgery. The use of anesthesia had a downside—the risk of cardiac arrest. As pharmacology and technology, such as defibrillators, developed, patient's hearts could be successfully restarted. Sometimes this was accomplished with minimal damage and a return to a high quality of life. At other times extensive damage occurred to individuals' neurological capabilities, leaving them comatose. Frequently, another arrest would cause death.

Difficulties arise in healthcare institutions because CPR can be performed by anyone who is properly trained. As a result, almost all patients or residents in a long term care setting, assuming the available technology, will have CPR performed whether or not it is of value, unless specific directions are given not to resuscitate them. This capability raises a variety of ethical issues regarding patient preferences and patient autonomy, the benefit of CPR for individual patients, the patient's ability to accept or reject any resuscitation, the cost of care, and appropriate decision makers. As of Jan. 1, 1988, the Joint Commission on Accreditation of Healthcare Organizations (JCAHO) requires hospital policy to spell out problems for do-not-resuscitate orders (DNR), to identify the operative principles, and to designate a committee that will help resolve differences about DNR orders.

Patient Issues

The first ethical issue is how to involve patients in a decision to resuscitate or not to resuscitate. On one hand, some argue that individuals who are critically ill or seriously compromised are incompetent to be involved in a DNR decision. To attempt to involve them in this decision will cause harm. On the other hand, others argue that patients, regardless of their critically ill status, can benefit from a decision-making discussion because of the finality of a DNR order.

The two sides of the ethical issue are (1) whether disclosure makes participation impossible because of the fear and conflict that it creates in the patient, or (2) whether not disclosing threatens the autonomy and values of the patient, thereby denying the benefits that would accrue to the patient by participating in the decision.

Another ethical issue is when to involve patients in a CPR discussion. Some argue that if individuals are unlikely to experience cardiac arrest, then raising these issues causes needless worry. For example, a patient admitted for an appendectomy might not need to be confronted with the question of resuscitation because cardiac arrest is unlikely to occur. On the other hand, individuals who are critically ill, who suffer from heart disease, or who have multiple organ system failure need to have the issue addressed.

Arguments are made from both sides; the issue is which values to promote. Should it be benefit, absolute autonomy, or full disclosure? Is information given at the discretion of the provider, or is full disclosure always required, even if cardiac arrest is a remote possibility? However, the issues must be discussed before cardiac arrest occurs. Once a person's heart has stopped, any delay in resuscitating the individual reduces the probable success of the resuscitation attempt. There will be no time for committee discussion or team interchange once an arrest has occurred. Thus, the issue must be raised before the time of arrest. But for whom?

This indicates the need for policies about DNR orders. Long term care facilities, although less likely to resuscitate residents than acute care hospitals, are no different in their obligation to this need. Each institution must address this problematic concern.

Benefits

Another ethical issue is what benefit CPR actually provides. Studies indicate that widespread use of CPR, for all patients, results in many resuscitative attempts with few patients successfully resuscitated and fewer returning home.[1] This difficulty indicates the need for patient selection for CPR and careful analysis of resuscitative attempts. Carefully selecting individuals who may benefit from CPR will help to ensure quality care and prevent individuals from unduly suffering from resuscitative attempts that should not take place. From an ethical perspective, the presumption is to favor resuscitative attempts, since its delay could create serious harm for a patient. This also requires decisions for DNR before an arrest occurs.

Other arguments are raised about the difficulty of knowing, with certainty, who will benefit or not benefit from CPR. One has to remember that trying to estimate the benefit of the procedure is a question of prudential judgment and not a question of certainty. Uncertainty about a successful outcome of CPR does not make the resuscitative attempt worthless, or a DNR order unethical. Certainty is not the moral issue. Benefit, as determined in the physician-patient relationship, is the moral issue.

Another ethical issue involving benefit is quality care. The discussion of quality of life is generally suspect because of subjectivity. Individuals fear that in some circumstances arbitrary decisions will be made to extend or to terminate treatment. Some persons respond to quality of life concerns by eliminating the issue of quality of life from the discussion. The difficulty with the elimination of quality of life criterion is that this criterion is a significant factor in the value-related choices that individuals make. Clarification about what one means by quality of life, sacredness of life, and sanctity of life are necessary in both CPR and DNR orders.

Costs

Another related ethical concern is cost. Cost is a factor in procedures that provide benefit, but it is almost never raised, especially when the benefit may be the patient's return to the home or to a continuation of life at a quality level acceptable to the patient. Some will argue that costs for continued aggressive resuscitation are not great. Others argue that unless one is certain of favorable outcomes, these expenditures are a poor use of societal resources.

Cost issues are difficult to assess because it is hard to know at what point a patient will experience cardiac arrest and need CPR. Since there are many different forms of cardiac arrest, the cost factor is further complicated. Some cardiac problems can be reversed with simple defibrillation or other aggressive measures. Other types of cardiac problems, complicated by other organ failure, may not respond to resuscitative attempts. These issues are impossible to predict.

The ethical issues of cost to society are also numerous. It is not difficult to imagine that society, insurance companies, and other third-party payers may decide to continue or refuse payment based on whether or not an individual agrees to a DNR order. In addition, DNR orders taken out of context can be used to imply the cessation of other treatment methods that the individual may desire. These social problems are especially pertinent in a time of limited resources and cost-containing strategies. The outcome in terms of beneficial care for patients will be compromised if cost is allowed to have too significant a role in this decision.

Decision Makers

A variety of problems arise concerning decision makers in a DNR order. Some argue that the decision is the prerogative of the physician since the physician knows "best." Others argue that patients should make the decision because respect for autonomy is a fundamental and primary ethical principle of healthcare delivery. Still others argue for a joint decision-making process that involves the physician and the patient. Ethical arguments are raised about nurses and other healthcare professionals frequently being more aware of the competent patient's wishes and the incompetent patient's family's wishes about medical treatment than physicians who see the patient only for short periods. Therefore, these other providers should be involved in decisions as well.

Decision makers for DNR orders are no different from any other medical decision makers. Respect for the clinical relationship and the mutuality factors of an established physician-patient relationship should be respected. There will always be a place for outside assistance from individuals who know the patient and from other medical team members.

Incompetent patients present more difficulties. Who should make decisions for the incompetent patient, and with what standards? The patient's expressed values? Standards determined by the person's best interests, as determined by the medical community? Or someone else's values?

The ethical debate about decision makers must consider all these issues. What is the appropriate role of the physician, the nurse, and other team members? Are there instances when the appropriate roles of those individuals are allowed to overcome the firmly established preferences and autonomy that a patient has?

Policies

These questions are resolved particularly well by institutional policies.[2] Providers discussing the need for policy point to experiences where the lack of policy led to poor decisions. Policies that were not written, written in shorthand, and not available to everyone, as well as cryptic statements such as "slow code," "chemical code only," and "no intubation," leave areas of ambiguity that should not exist in DNR orders. These and other experiences have forced people to ask questions about how best to develop policies.

From an ethical perspective, clearly stated policies help deliver patient care that respects the autonomy of individuals. Clear policies also ensure effective communication so all team members know what the appropriate response is to an individual who experiences cardiac arrest. Policies will also provide an opportunity for caregivers to have the latitude necessary to make decisions at the moment of arrest. As a result, people who want to be coded can have codes stopped after these have been initiated when it becomes clear that continued aggressive treatment is futile.

Sound policies also address ambiguous ethical issues such as whether or not to provide the opportunity for a DNR order when the resuscitative attempt might be futile. Another question that needs addressing is what the CPR or DNR order means. If individuals say that they wish to be resuscitated should cardiac arrest occur, does this indicate that they are arguing for these aggressive medical treatments in all circumstances? If patients indicate that they do not wish to be resuscitated and want a DNR order placed on their chart, does this mean that all aggressive medical treatment should cease? Is it possible to contend, as some do, that resuscitative attempts mean simply that individuals should not be resuscitated should cardiac arrest occur, but should be treated for other problems such as pneumonia or other treatable problems?

Some even raise questions about what the general patient care plan should be if a DNR order is written. If a DNR order is written, does it indicate that acute care is no longer appropriate? Does this mean that the individual should be moved from an intensive care unit to another unit? Does a DNR order mean that the individual should be moved from the acute care institution to a different level of care, perhaps a hospice, where palliation and care will continue, but aggressive treatments will not be given?

Conclusion

Many questions are raised by DNR orders. Although the technology provides an opportunity for a "second" life for some individuals when appropriately applied, it also can continue life with an individual in a vegetative state, waiting for death to occur from still another arrest at a later time. The ethical issues surrounding DNR orders are not unlike ethical issues in any other life-sustaining issues of medicine where ambiguity and confusion arise and require clarification through careful reasoning.

1. S. Bedell et al., "Survival after Cardiopulmonary Resuscitation in the Hospital," *New England Journal of Medicine* 10:309, 1983, pp. 569–576.
2. *Accreditation Manual for Hospitals 1988,* Joint Commission on Accreditation of Hospitals, Chicago, 1988, pp. 90–91.

Advanced Directives: Living Wills and Durable Power of Attorney Acts

Institutional ethics committees, acute care hospitals, and long term care facilities have had to deal with an increasing number of living will or natural death acts passed by state legislatures over the last 10 years. Institutions in states that have not passed living wills still grapple with the issue as remaining states address this type of legislation, as they take an active role in promoting or defeating proposed advance directives, or as patients and residents present personally executed documents that request the withholding or withdrawing of certain types of medical treatment.

Living wills as legal documents were first introduced in a "Natural Death Act" in the state of California in 1976. This initial legislation and the acts that followed attempt to provide individuals, who may later be incompetent and incapable of directing their healthcare, an opportunity to state their preferences for treatment. This was done for three reasons. The first is that technology extending an individual's life for a long period continues to develop. If the extension of one's life resulted in an active return to society, questions would not be raised. However, technology sometimes extends physiological existence with minimal cognitive or conscious activity.

The second reason is the rise of the importance of patient autonomy. As the saga of Karen Ann Quinlan gained national attention, people sought avenues to allow them to stop unwanted medical treatments. If competent, a person is allowed to refuse any medical treatment. When incompetent, there is no guarantee that personal values will be respected. Thus, attempts were made to provide specific directions in this situation.

The third reason is the legal uncertainty of withholding or withdrawing so-called life-saving medical interventions. Institutions and physicians seek protection from the courts, whereas patients and their families seek to assert their rights. Presently, a few states have not passed some type of advance directive that allows individuals either to specify treatments they would or would not want or to choose a decision maker to make choices for them should they become incompetent.

Types of Advance Directives

There are two types of advance directives. The first is a directive designed to give information to the incompetent patient about which treatments are acceptable or unacceptable; the second identifies the decision maker for the incompetent patient.

The first is usually known as a "living will," as a "natural death act," or by euphemisms used to describe directions for withholding or withdrawing treatment from incompetent persons. These directives are made when the patient is competent and able to express clear statements about his or her choices for future healthcare. Living wills come in a variety of forms, and no uniform "living will act" is applicable in all states. Each state has designed its own statute adding certain specifications that restrict when, what, and how a living will can be executed.

The second type of advance directive is modeled after a "durable power of attorney act," a legal mechanism that allows an individual to appoint another person to make a legally binding decision when one is not physically present to do this oneself. An individual leaving a particular area or state can specify another person to carry out legal or contractual obligations on his or her behalf. A durable power of attorney act for healthcare decisions is an attempt to allow individuals to appoint specific decision makers to make healthcare decisions once those individuals are incompetent.

Both types of advance directives are designed to safeguard and protect the person affected by the decision maker and to have decisions made in accordance with personal values.

The Values and Disvalues of Advance Directives

Many individuals promote the idea of living wills. First, they argue that individuals have a right to make decisions about the acceptance or rejection of any medical treatment based on their right to privacy and self-determination. When an individual becomes incompetent to make these decisions, these rights still exist and should be respected. A living will is a method to protect the patient's right of self-determination. By identifying what the patient wants or does not want through a living will, executed when the person is competent, the individual's autonomy is respected.

Second, respecting a person's living will shows respect for the person. Respecting the self-determination of an individual while competent should be carried out when he or she is incompetent. Honoring a living will is one way of continuing this respect for the person. The living will provides information to the physician, other caregivers, and the family about what decisions would have been made by the patient if he or she were still competent.

Not all people, however, agree with this assessment. Some people have problems with living will legislation in general or with the specifics of a legislative attempt in an individual state. First, they argue that living wills promote dying rather than living. Since society does not want to protect vulnerable individuals or respect those individuals whose "quality of life" or whose "productivity" in life is not "acceptable," living wills provide one more mechanism by which a "death culture" rather than a "life culture" flourishes. Those who oppose living wills state that society should promote the life of vulnerable patients more aggressively.

Second, they point to the uncertainty of a living will's validity at the time of implementing the specific directives. Other people question the validity of the living will itself. Questions are raised about whether or not the incompetent patient was competent when the living will was executed. Others question the validity of the living will in regard to how it reflects the state statute and the meaning of the law. Further, questions are raised about whether or not the patient was aware and conscious of all the qualifications and ramifications of signing the living will. Would an individual in a healthy state understand the complexities and problems of being ill, especially being ill at the end of life? Consequently, the validity of a living will, although duly executed, is questioned from a variety of angles.

Frequently, living wills specify what can be asked for or refused. A prime example is artificial nutrition and hydration. Increasingly, living wills prevent people from requesting the withdrawal or withholding of any type of nutrition or hydration based on the assumption that artificial nutrition and hydration are basic human care and do not fall into the category of extraordinary, useless, or burdensome treatment.

Other examples of particular therapies can be cited. However, the primary issue remains the same. A focus on therapies rather than personal values is generally unhelpful.

Problems of Living Wills in General

Each state's living will statute has problems. Limitations are involved in respecting the wishes of individual incompetent patients. Living wills are restricted only to those who suffer from terminal diseases and are imminently dying. A living will can be implemented only when the individual fulfills all these criteria.

This poses numerous difficulties. First, individuals who are terminally ill, incompetent, and imminently dying will die whether or not life-sustaining treatments are applied. The living will does nothing to either prolong the life or shorten the dying process of these individuals. Yet, in most states, living wills are designed to refute or end treatment only in these circumstances.

The second problem is that most living will legislation, although attempting to secure the rights of the incompetent patient, also allows individual physicians and providers to focus on validity issues. The living will is not accepted as a valid document. Attempts to refute the directions of the individual's advance directive are made until the physician or institution proves the document's validity. One understands the desire of institutions and healthcare providers to promote life. Nonetheless, the promotion of life that denies the patient's wishes to forego certain types of medical treatment violates the very values the living will tries to promote.

The third problem is the questioning of the patient's comprehensive knowledge at the time the living will was executed. Could the individual have a clear awareness of what could physically debilitate them and what the implications of given therapies are for a future medical problem? If the answer to that question is no, then the living will could not be valid.

The last problem involves the limitations on the forms of treatments that can or cannot be accepted within the context of a living will. If a living will restricts the individual's ability to accept or reject certain treatments, such as artificial nutrition and hydration, then the individual's right to make choices for himself or herself is compromised. The issue extends to many other issues, such as administration of antibiotics or other types of care that provide no benefit for the individual when he or she is dying or critically ill. The attempt to limit specific medical interventions does not recognize the complex and ambiguous setting in which medical therapies are provided and medical decisions made. The focus is on the particular treatment, and not on the patient's values.

Other Problems

The most difficult problems of medical decision making involve the critically ill, incompetent patient who is not "terminally ill" and "imminently dying." As noted, individuals who are incompetent, terminally ill, and imminently dying die regardless of technology. How should one treat the critically ill patient who could live for some period, anywhere from weeks to months, but who would die in a relatively short time if certain treatments were stopped? Does a living will have force for this patient? Can individuals choose to forego certain types of medical treatment that may prolong their physiological life or their physiological and minimally conscious life for a short or long period? Can someone refuse treatments and be allowed to die soon when continued medical treatments could continue life for an extended time? How does one account for the burden of treatment or the values of a person in these situations? A question that faces most hospitals and long term care facilities is how to balance particular treatments and personal values for the incompetent patient who is critically ill but not dying soon.

To resolve this dilemma, several ethical and medical issues must be addressed. The first is the concept of *burdens* associated with treatment. Burdens fall into various categories. One is the context of pain or difficulty associated with administering a particular treatment; another is the cost of the treatment. One category involves the emotional and related difficulties that the individual's family may experience. The point is not that family burdens necessarily override the individual's continued treatment but that family burdens are considered part of the patient's perception of burdens. In many circumstances, individuals do not want family members to carry economic burdens for treatments that continue life at minimal levels. In all circumstances, burdens involve the patient's ability to pursue life's goals and values. Burdens are not measured only for terminally ill, imminently dying patients, but rather are a part of all medical decision making.

The second problem is the technological possibility of maintaining physiological life alone. Medical technology provides an opportunity to maintain a person's physiological life for months and years despite a permanent loss of consciousness. Paul Brophy, Karen Ann Quinlan, and others illustrate this problem. Just because medicine can maintain a person's physiological existence for an extended period does not mean that continued medical intervention is a value. Nonetheless, most living wills are not honored in these circumstances.

A third difficulty is the wide array of treatments available to people suffering from critical illnesses that might not be accepted by the competent individual. If one works on the assumption that competent patients are able to refuse medical treatment that is too burdensome or useless, it is difficult to understand why the same treatment cannot be refused by incompetents patients through an advanced directive. No religious sect or philosophical group holds firmly to the belief that the maintenance of solely physiological life is an ultimate value. Society needs to protect human life. However, respecting physiological life alone is not good medicine or good ethics.

Lastly, if living wills are to be of any use at all, then legislation must address what is meant by the term *extraordinary care*. Extraordinary care cannot be defined by a particular medical therapy or intervention. Rather, extraordinary care is a measure of the benefits and burdens, the usefulness and uselessness of a particular treatment for an individual patient in accordance with his or her personal values. Granted, this is very difficult to put into law. Individual institutions and providers, however, must deal with this ambiguous situation if advance directives are to have meaning.

Durable Power of Attorney Acts for Healthcare Decisions

The central issue of advance directives is the ability of individuals to communicate personal values and choices for the delivery of healthcare when they are no longer competent. Preferably, individuals will discuss with healthcare providers their personal preferences while competent. When such discussion cannot take place, and when advance directives do not allow for clarification of what is valued or not valued in continued treatment, then the need arises to identify a proxy decision maker to make decisions for the incompetent person.

Durable power of attorney acts for healthcare decisions are a more prudent avenue for this decision making. A durable power of attorney allows an individual to identify a proxy decision maker whom he or she trusts to express his or her values and to discuss with the institution or healthcare provider what treatments are appropriate and inappropriate.

Developing legislative statutes to extend durable power of attorney acts, which exist in all states, to encompass healthcare decision making in low-cost, easy-to-implement fashion is a legislative priority. The durable power of attorney act for healthcare decisions provides a guarantee that there will be partners in a communicative setting within the institution or within the patient-provider relationship to discuss and explore the various alternatives available in medicine. As institutions deal with this issue, they need to address the concerns of the terminally ill, imminently dying patient (who is going to die regardless of what is done), as well as the concerns of incompetent individuals whose illness is critical (but the person is not imminently dying) and who would question continued treatment.

Only a few states have established durable power of attorney acts for healthcare matters. These states have either had "living wills" and sought something better suited to decision making or decided that a durable power of attorney act is a better route than living wills. These state statutes and experiences may be helpful for other states considering this type of legislation.

Conclusions

There is little doubt that the movement toward advance directives will continue. Two important considerations should be noted. First, the identification of individuals who can enter into a meaningful and competent dialogue with physicians and institutions about the needs, values, and wishes of an incompetent patient will always be more helpful than written documents. The difficulty is how to identify appropriate proxies.

Second, the principles of allowing to die provide a background of information not presently available in advance directive legislation. It is not only the terminally ill, incompetent, and imminently dying patient who needs to have a mechanism to remove certain types of medical treatment; it is also the critically ill patient for whom continued treatment is too burdensome. The ambiguity of "burdensomeness" as a criterion needs to be discussed and developed further for advance directives to be helpful in the increasingly complex and technological setting of contemporary medicine.

Nancy Beth Cruzan: A Case of 29
Proxy Consent

In southwest Missouri, Nancy Beth Cruzan lies unconscious in a state hospital in a persistent vegetative state. Although her family and several religious and ethical advisors believe it is time to allow Nancy to die, their decision may not be implemented. Instead, her fate is being determined by the courts of Missouri. Severely injured five years ago in an automobile accident, Nancy never regained consciousness. Medical experts called to testify offer different technical explanations of her condition, but all agree that she will not regain the potential to function in a cognitive-affective manner.

Given the ineffective application of medical therapy and the burden resulting from the use of life-prolonging devices, Nancy's parents have requested that all therapy be removed from their daughter. The Missouri attorney general is contesting the Cruzan's request, maintaining that removal of life support would amount to murder. Judge Charles Teel determined at the trial court level that life support in the form of artificial nutrition and hydration could be removed because these are medical means to prolong life and are no longer effective. In November 1988, the Supreme Court of Missouri, in a decision highly criticized for legal and ethical reasons, overruled the trial court and mandated that artificial hydration and nutrition be continued.

In this essay, we are not so much concerned with the decisions of the Missouri courts; rather we wish to consider more basic issues. Why do we devote so much attention to the medical treatment of people who are unable to speak for themselves? When should the authority of the courts supplant the decisions of the family members? What norms should parents, guardians, or officials of the court follow when making decisions for medical care of seriously debilitated people? The Cruzan case prompts the study of the ethical values and norms involved in proxy and surrogate consent.

The Principles

Incompetent persons, whether conscious or unconscious, cannot make ethical decisions for themselves. Incompetence arises from different causes and may be partial or total. Thus, a person may be competent to make decisions about daily wants and needs, but incompetent to manage property. In this essay, we are concerned with incompetency that is total because of physical or mental deprivation, and we focus on the decisions concerning medical care that such deprivation necessitates.

No matter what the condition of an incompetent person, he or she is still a human being and is to be treated as a person. In recognition of each human person's worth and value, no matter how debilitated or moribund the person might be, society recognizes that the incompetent person must be given care that will protect the person's dignity as a human being. To facilitate the proper care for incompetent persons, society recognizes that competent persons must speak for incompetent ones. The recognition that incompetent people should have a proxy or surrogate speak for them when important human needs are in question is cross-cultural. That is, proxy consent is one of the ethical norms found in all types of civilizations and cultures.

Usually, a family member is called on to act as proxy for the incompetent person. Family members are considered most apt to fulfill the role of proxy or surrogate because of the presumption that family members love one another and will act in the best interests of the incompetent family member. Again, this presumption that family members should act as surrogates is cross-cultural. However, if it seems that family members are about to make decisions that are not beneficial for the incompetent person, or if a serious ethical dilemma exists concerning the proper action to be performed on behalf of the incompetent person, then the power of the civil law may be invoked to make a decision. Clearly, if the family's responsibilities to act as proxy are to be superseded by the courts, there must be evidence either that the family members are not acting in the best interests of the incompetent person, or that the proper medical treatment for the person is uncertain. Involving the court to appoint a guardian if there is no evidence of malfeasance or a serious ethical dilemma is a violation of the bonds of love and the ethical presumptions on which a peaceful society is based. What right do the courts have to interfere in family affairs when matters are determined justly and peacefully?

What goal should the proxy decision maker have in mind when making decisions for an incompetent person? Should the proxy seek to determine which actions will prolong life? Or should the proxy ask what is most beneficial for the incompetent person? Should the proxy be held to do what the incompetent person would have done were he or she able to make a decision? In the United States, the courts and most ethicists maintain that because persons are autonomous, they have a right to be treated as they would wish were they capable of making a decision. Thus, the prior wishes of the incompetent patient are often presented as an absolute norm for proxy decision making. For two reasons, however, this norm seems flawed. First, the proxy may not have a definite idea of what the incompetent person would have decided. Second, if the incompetent person has made known his or her desires, it may require that he or she be put to death by means of a lethal injection if ever in a persistent vegetative state. Fulfilling such a request would be unethical on the part of the proxy.

Discussion

A better ethical norm seems to be that the proxy should choose what a reasonable person would decide in the same circumstances. This norm applies whether or not the proxy knows the prior wishes of the incompetent person. If the person's wishes are known, they become the first informational source for this "reasonable decision." If the known wishes are ethical, then they should be given predominant consideration in forming the final decision. The second informational source for the proxy decision when the wishes are known is the effect that a particular decision will have on other people. The incompetent person, having made the decision concerning terminal care, would not know all the circumstances existing when the decision is actually applied. If prolonging the life of an incompetent person would require round-the-clock nursing care plus depletion of a family's savings and loss of their home and livelihood, would a "reasonable person" determine to have his or her life prolonged? Or if withdrawing care would endanger a person's spiritual destiny, would a "reasonable person" withdraw care?

In our era, people seek to ensure proxy decisions in accord with their wishes through living wills and durable power of attorney. Both instruments are insufficient for the task at hand. First, legal documents remove decision making concerning medical care from loved ones. Second, in making decisions concerning the care of a debilitated person, so many variables exist that they could not all be envisioned in a legal document. Clearly, it behooves family members to discuss beforehand the type of care they would prefer when incapacitated and in need of life support. To imagine, however, that the ethical requests of a person are valid only if verified by legal document belittles the bonds of love and trust that preserve society.

Conclusion

The effort to determine in a court of law the proper care of a totally incompetent person who will never regain consciousness is subject to question. Why do loving parents need the approval of the courts to perform an ethical action? Have we become so litigious in our society that no distinction exists between law and ethics? Or has technology incapacitated the ability of elected officials to recognize what constitutes beneficial medical treatment? Whatever the cause, it seems the wrong people are offering proxy consent for Nancy Beth Cruzan.

King Solomon and Baby M   30

In New Jersey two couples contested in court the custody of an infant whose existence would have been unlikely 10 years ago. Conceived by Mary Beth Whitehead from the sperm of William Stern, which was introduced into her body through artificial insemination, the infant was given the name Sara by her maternal parents and Melissa by her paternal parents. She was named Baby M by the media.

Artificial insemination is nothing new. The novel and complicating issue in this case is that Mary Beth Whitehead after promising to give her baby to the Sterns immediately after birth, changed her mind and wished to rear the child in her family. Thus, not only does this case present some novel questions about custody of children, the question arises whether to recognize legally contracts for so-called surrogate motherhood. A more accurate term for the contract is *surrogate parenting* because the father is a surrogate as well. As happens so often in our society, the contestants in this dispute went to court to solve an ethical issue. At present, however, no laws and no court decisions offer guidance for an ethical solution.

Principles

As noted in an earlier essay, an intimate relationship exists between ethics and law, but one discipline does not substitute for the other. Ethics is a more fundamental and wide-reaching discipline; it concerns private as well as public behavior. Law concerns public behavior and is designed to establish justice by protecting ethical relationships in public life. Thus, the decisions of courts and legislatures should be based on ethical norms. The need for ethical investigation before new laws or new decisions of courts are rendered is obvious. If there is no such investigation, then our public policy will be built on faulty foundations.

What ethical norms should have governed the court decision in the case of Baby M? Should custody have been granted on the grounds that enforcing contracts is an ethical responsibility of the courts? If so, it seems the Sterns should have received custody. Should the ethical perspective of maternal relationship to the child have been emphasized? If so, the decision would seemingly have been in favor of the Whiteheads. Should the decision have been based on the predicted benefits that Baby M would experience living in either home? Determining ethical norms on the basis of this perspective demands not only predictions about the future, but, also a determination of which parental qualities truly benefit a child. (See postscript at the end of the essay.)

Several pundits had observed that Justice Harvey Sorkow would have to be a new King Solomon to solve the case of Baby M equitably and ethically. Let us study the famous decision of King Solomon to see if it provides any ethical insight for the solution to this case.

Two women came before King Solomon with a dispute (1 Kings 3:16). Both women lived in the same house, and each had a child. One of the children died in the night, and each mother claimed the living infant as her own. King Solomon, called on to decide which was the true mother, ordered that the living child should be cut in half and a half given to each mother. Obviously, it was only a symbolic solution by King Solomon, but the solution prompted action. One woman was prepared to accept the decision even if it should mean the death of the child; the other rejected the decision even though it meant losing the custody of the child who would continue to live. King Solomon declared the woman willing to surrender her claim to the child to save the child's life to be the true mother.

Why did the King decide in this manner? True motherhood is not possessive. A mother, in the valid sense of the word, does not act as though her child belongs to her; rather, she considers the life and well-being of her child more important than her own. The actions we value in motherhood are actions that bespeak life, generosity, and enabling love, not actions that connote ownership, domination, or commerce.

Discussion

The lessons from King Solomon's decision are valid today. Children are never to be considered as possessions of their parents. No one has a right to buy or own children. We may have a right to certain basic needs that are necessary to live a decent life, such as a right to food, housing, education, and healthcare. But no one has a right to a child. First and fundamentally, a child is not a possession or property. Second, children are not to be used by parents to improve their own prospects in life. Bringing children into the world is a gift of life to another human being, not an investment directed toward the satisfaction of parents. The basis for parent-child relationships is not a limiting legal contract, but rather a mutual act of love. This act of mutual love perdures after birth and ensures that the child will be respected and reared as a person, not raised as a possession. Parenting of human beings should be characterized by continuing generosity and self-sacrifice if the child generated is to have an opportunity to live as a free and responsible human being.

Parenthood is not a commercial enterprise nor a transitory commitment. Thus, when a woman agrees to conceive and bear a child for someone other than her husband, she is treating the child to be conceived as a possession, something she is free to give away or sell. When a father contracts to supply sperm for conception of a child, he engages in fabricating a product, not in an act of love. If fecundation occurs and the woman cooperates, the father will have a new possession that he is free to keep, or discard if it seems flawed.

Moreover, the family is a cause as well as a result of evolutionary development.[1] If we legalize the process of renting wombs and buying children, we act contrary to three million years of evolution. Finally, through surrogate parenting, we ask women to act directly contrary to the values associated with responsible motherhood, since this form of parenting demands that mothers be prepared *not* to love their children.

Conclusion

For these serious reasons, it seems that Judge Sorkow and other justices and legislatures across the United States should declare "surrogate motherhood" illegal because it is unethical.

Simply because a novel form of fertilization and gestation is possible does not imply that it is ethical, nor does it imply that it should become public policy.

Postscript

On March 31, 1987, Judge Sorkow awarded custody of Baby M to William Stern, the biological father, and stripped the mother Mary Beth Whitehead, of all parental rights. The judge upheld the surrogate mother contract and dismissed all arguments that the contract violated state adoption laws and public policies against the sale of babies. After reading his three-hour decision, Judge Sorkow permitted Elizabeth Stern to legally adopt Baby M.

On appeal, the Supreme Court of New Jersey, on Feb. 3, 1988, allowed the Sterns to retain custody of Baby M. By a unanimous decision, however, the court overturned all other aspects of the Sorkow decision. The ruling restored parental visitation rights of the baby's mother, reversing the permission of Elizabeth Stern to adopt the child. Finally, the surrogate contract was declared invalid because it conflicts with law and public policy and is illegal, and perhaps criminal, as well as potentially degrading to women.[2]

1. Donald C. Johanson and Maitland Edey, *Lucy: The Beginnings of Human Kind,* Warner Books, New York, 1982.
2. See *The New York Times,* March 31, 1987, to Feb. 3, 1988.

Baby Doe Regulations 31

In June 1986, the U.S. Supreme Court made a decision invalidating the federal regulations designed to require life-prolonging medical treatment for severely handicapped infants. The regulations that the Supreme Court overruled were known as the "Baby Doe Regs." These rules were initially established because of the experience of a child with Down's syndrome born in Bloomington, IN, with esophageal atresia. Baby Doe's parents decided not to allow surgery to clear the blockage in his esophagus and allow him to live. Their decision was based on his having Down's syndrome.

Shortly after that, Baby Jane Doe was born in Long Island, NY, with spina bifida. Her parents made the decision to treat her medically rather than surgically and to take her home. In part their decision reflected concerns not about life and death, but about which treatment provided the best quality of life for their child.

These two cases, and others similar to them, raise questions about what the appropriate decision-making processes should be when dealing with impaired infants.

Court Decisions

A few months after the Baby Doe issue arose, the federal government mandated certain regulations through the Department of Health and Human Services (DHHS) to secure appropriate care for all children born with life-threatening impairments. Three different regulations would be promulgated by the DHHS; each would be challenged in the court, either for procedural reasons or because of their contents.

The federal government tried to obtain the medical records of Baby Jane Doe under one set of these regulations, only to find the attempt blocked by New York state courts. This ruling was appealed to the U.S. Supreme Court. The court ruled on this appeal. Primarily, the ruling denied the ability of the federal government to access Baby Jane Doe's records to check whether or not she was treated appropriately.

Decision Making

The Supreme Court may have provided a "legal out" from the Baby Doe Regulations, and it may secure the right of privacy of the American people in making healthcare decisions, but the ethical issues still remain. The legal ruling will have a limited impact on the ethical concerns that healthcare institutions, physicians, parents, and children confront. Each institution that deals with impaired infants must continue to face the ethical questions of decision making.

A first issue is the value of life. Life has always been perceived as the greatest value. Without physical life, it becomes impossible to pursue any other human values. Questions arise when further distinctions are made about the quality of life and/or the sanctity of life. Although one upholds the *sanctity* of each person's life, meaning that each person's life is respected, one also has to ask questions about the *quality* of life. Balancing sanctity and quality is a critical issue. Sole emphasis on sanctity can lead to a vitalist position, whereas arbitrary emphasis on quality can lead to disrespect for ill, impaired, or aged persons.

A second ethical issue is the principle of proxy consent. More than in other areas of medicine, neonatal medicine points to the time-consuming process that consent involves. To consent to a procedure, one needs to know what is wrong. It is important for providers to have adequate time for an accurate diagnosis and prognosis. Very young children are unable to participate in the medical examination by helping providers to understand what is wrong or what they are feeling. Diagnostic work can be more time consuming. Newborns can experience complications that manifest themselves only after a certain period. In addition, trying to understand the impact of an impairment on a child and the child's future is not done quickly. As a result, if decisions are made previous to these time-consuming diagnostic workups, the decisons are likely to be poor.

Family discussion is a necessary element of the consent process. Not infrequently, a woman may be hospitalized in one institution while her child is transferred to a high-level tertiary-care neonatal institution in another city. In addition, a father, if present, has other family and work obligations that take him away from the day-to-day, moment-to-moment decision process. The distance that separates mother, father, and child makes consensus decision making difficult. As a result, waiting for families to gather, for mothers to be discharged from other institutions, and for the family to participate in the decision-making process takes time.

Also, the consent issues require a consensual dialogue between physicians and parents. One of the weaknesses of the Baby Doe Regulations is the belief that regulations can take care of the intricate decision-making process. The consensual dialogue needs to occur in a clinical setting rather than at a committee meeting. Value-based decisions are the result of time and relationships, not regulations.

Death and Dying

The third ethical issue is allowing to die. Everyone dies, and unfortunately some die as infants, denied the ability to pursue the purposes and goals of life. Although life-saving technologies in the neonatal unit may provide an opportunity to perform many aspects of care for children, the presence of the neonatal institution does not guarantee life itself. Two questions must be asked in this area. The first is, how useful or useless are the treatments available? For some children, such as those who suffer from hypoplastic left-sided heart syndrome, for example, no known therapy exists to correct the life-threatening problem. As a result, the pursuit of high-tech medicine may prolong the child's dying and not the child's living. There is no moral obligation to perform useless treatments.

More difficult to assess, however, is the second question. How burdened can a child be and still have life? How does respect for the sanctity of each child's life affect the decision-making process when it comes to administering therapeutic measures that are highly burdensome, that leave the child institutionalized apart from family contact, or that prevent the child from being able to ever touch or feel the outside world. Ethically, no one is obliged to accept burdensome treatment when burdensome is defined in relation to the infant's ability to pursue the goals of life, and when the goal of life is defined as more than the maintenance of physical life only.

Finally, each institution must address the issue of team work. The best medicine is done in teams, and this is also true in neonatology. The constant presence of the nurse, the need for many subspecialists to make an accurate diagnosis and to treat the child effectively, the ability of pastoral care and social workers to work hand-in-hand with the emotional needs of families, and the capacity to help families make prudent decisions for their children point to this reality. No one physician is able to manage all this. The physician is still the team leader and helps orchestrate the work for the child's benefit, but it is the team that accomplishes the healthcare goals.

Conclusion

Although the U.S. Supreme Court's decision may end another chapter of the "Baby Doe Regs" and preclude the government from having access to a child's records, it does not resolve the difficult ethical issues. Ethics committees, some form of infant-care review committee, or another forum within a healthcare institution must address these ethical issues if appropriate care is to be rendered to neonates.

Anencephaly, Brain Death,   32
and Transplants

In response to a shortage of kidneys for transplant into children, a medical team in West Germany has initiated the practice of removing kidneys from anencephalic infants.[1] The infants are intubated immediately on birth and given ventilator support. The kidneys are then removed and transplanted. The medical team announces that the transplants are successful. But, of course, the donor dies because vital organs have been removed. The medical team argues that anencephalic infants should "be considered brain dead." Moreover, they maintain that "the anencephalic fetus because of the absence of brain development has never been alive despite the presence of heart beat." The main justification offered by the transplant team for securing organs in this manner is that the federal courts in West Germany and the United States allow the abortion of anencephalic infants.

Is there any scientific justification for maintaining that anencephalic infants are brain dead? Is there any ethical justification for treating anencephalic infants, or other severely debilitated infants who will soon die, as though they were already dead?

Anencephaly

Anencephaly is the congenital absence of the cranial vault, with the cerebral hemispheres completely missing or reduced to small masses. It results from a defect in the closure at the anterior portion of the neural groove. The malformation results in a severely underdeveloped, or undeveloped, cerebral cortex. However, the brainstem, or lower brain, does develop and integrates digestion, respiration, and other human functions, at least for a short time if the infant is born alive. Many fetuses with anencephaly are stillborn or die shortly after birth. The longest documented survival of an anencephalic infant has been five and a half months. Advances in diagnostic ultrasound allow the reliable diagnosis of anencephaly before birth if the head can be adequately visualized.

What happens when vital organs, such as the kidneys, are removed from an anencephalic infant? As in the case of any other human being, death ensues when the vital organs are removed. The removal of the organs are the direct cause of death. Just as removing vital organs from a young or older person in irreversible coma would be a willful, direct, and premeditated cause of death, so removing the same organs would be a willful, direct, and premeditated cause of death for the anencephalic infant.

Criteria for Death

Would it be reasonable to consider an anencephalic infant dead simply because the cerebral cortex does not develop? One characteristic of living things that is absent in dead human beings is the body's capacity to organize and regulate itself. Death is that moment when the body's physiological system ceases to constitute a unified homeostatic system and becomes disorganized into a mere collection of heterogeneous chemical substances. After death, some cells or organs may continue for a time, perhaps indefinitely if artificially supported, to exhibit some life signs, but they are not the unified actions of a living being. To know that death has occurred, one must be reasonably sure of three things:

1. The body does not exhibit specific human behavior

2. The body will not be able to exhibit such behavior in the future

3. The body no longer has even a radical capacity for human functions because it has lost the basic structure required for human unity.

Although the function of some vital organs, such as the heart, lungs, and kidneys, have played an important part in determining death, the most fundamental element that separates life from death is the ability of the body to function as an integrated homeostatic unity. If time is not important, even the layperson can judge that another person is dead; after a time the dead body will loose all signs of life and begin to decay. For legal and medical reasons, however, a decision that death has occurred is usually required shortly after the event. Thus, medical science seeks clinical criteria to define and diagnose the death of an individual with greater celerity.

What role does the brain function have in establishing and maintaining integral human functions and thus in the determination of death? An extensive summary in regard to the clinical criteria for determining human death is found in *Defining Death*, the report of the President's Commission for the Study of Ethical Problems in Medicine and Biomedical and Behavioral Research.[2] In accord with traditional practice, the commission accepts irreversible cessation of spontaneous cardiopulmonary function as one clinical criterion for death. Thus, if the heart and lungs cease functioning and their function cannot be restored or supplemented, a person may be declared dead. The Commission, however, in accord with modern medical practice and philosophical theory, maintains that death also may be determined if brain function is lacking. Thus, there are not two forms of human death, but two sets of criteria exist for judging the occurrence of death. This second method of determining death is more germane to our discussion. For determination of human death using brain function as the criterion, the Commission requires cessation "of all functions of the entire brain including the brain stem." The Commission adds:

> This makes plain the intent to exclude from application under the definition any patient who has lost only higher brain functions or conversely who maintains those functions but has suffered solely a direct injury to the brainstem which interferes with the vegetative functions of the body.[3]

That "brain death" involves more than the higher brain function also was made clear in one of the first scientific seminars to investigate this topic. The seminar participants agreed that: "[B]rain death is defined as irreversible destruction of the neuronal contents of the intracranial cavity. This includes both cerebral hemispheres, including cortex and deep structures, as well as the brain stem and the cerebellum. An equivalent term is total brain infarction to the first cervical level of the spinal cord."[4]

Other Possible Criteria for Human Death

The President's Commission rejects explicitly the theory that higher brain death alone, that is, absence of function in the cortex with the brainstem retaining its function, would constitute a criterion for human death:

> At present, neither basic neurophysiology nor medical technique suffices to translate the "higher brain" formulation (of death) into policy. First . . . it is not known which portions of the brain are responsible for cognition and consciousness; what little is known points to substantial interconnections among brainstem, subcortical structures, and the neocortex. Thus, the "higher brain" may well exist only as a metaphorical concept, not in reality. Second, even when the sites of certain aspects of consciousness can be found, their cessation often cannot be assessed with the certainty that would be required in applying a statutory definition.[5]

If only higher brain function were assessed in determining death, it would violate our social values as well, since it would allow the burial of people while they are still breathing and pulsating spontaneously.

Some philosophers would maintain that an anencephalic infant is a human being but not a person. Using this distinction, they would allow procedures to be performed on a human being that they would not allow on a *person*. Does a distinction between human being and person allow anencephalic infants to be treated as though they were dead? Although a difference may exist in terms, no difference exists in rights insofar as the individual is concerned. As the President's Commission pointed out when rejecting this distinction, "crucial to the personhood argument is acceptance of one particular concept of those things that are essential to being a person while there is no general agreement on this very fundamental point."[6] Moreover, if one admits that a distinction of rights results from the terms *person* and *human being,* then the vital and inalienable rights of a person would stem from a grant from society rather than from existence as a human being. History indicates that discrimination, suffering, and death result from the concept, "The state grants inalienable rights."

Is there any scientific evidence that indicates that because an anencephalic infant does not develop a cerebral cortex, he or she is not a human being? Could development of the cerebral cortex be considered a "marker event" separating prehuman and human development? In 1985, when studying the matter of experimentation on human embryos, a select committee of the Parliament of the Commonwealth of Australia stated: "No marker ever advanced carried such weight that different principles should apply to distinguish the fertilized ovum from that which all would agree is a human subject."[7]

Thus, the Australian committee rejects as unscientific the notion that markers exist in the progressive development of an embryo, such as development of the primitive streak or the cerebral cortex, and enable one to determine that human life begins after fertilization. Although the anencephalic infant may not develop in a manner that fulfills the full potential usually associated with "person," there has never been a time when anencephalic infants were considered dead because their cerebral cortex had not developed. Rather, they have been considered as living human beings until their brainstem ceased to function.

Conclusion

Applying these scientific and social thoughts to the anencephalic infant, we conclude that when born, this infant is a living human being. True, he or she is a severely debilitated human being who will not live for long. But human beings prove their nobility by respecting the moral worth of the weak. Because there are no effective means of overcoming the pathology from which the anencephalic infant suffers, therapeutic care may be withheld. For this reason, an anencephalic infant rightly receives only comfort care because no moral obligation exists to try to prolong the life of such an infant as there is for most other infants. The real and dramatic difference between allowing a person to die because a serious pathology cannot be overcome and directly killing an innocent human being, however, mandates that anencephalic infants not be donors of human organs until after they are totally brain dead. Anticipating the death of the infant and keeping body fluids flowing after death through use of a respirator would not be unethical. The anencephalic infant could be treated in the same manner as an accident victim whose cerebral cortex has been severely injured, but whose brainstem has not ceased to function. But no organs should be removed until death has been certified from clinical signs.

Our era has a strong inclination to allow actions that are destructive if greater good is promised. This is especially true if weak persons are the victims. Experience and history indicate vividly, however, that we ultimately regret such actions.

1. Wolfgang Holzgreve et al., "Kidney Transplantation from Anencephalic Donors," *New England Journal of Medicine* 316:17, Apr. 23, 1987, pp. 1069–1070.
2. President's Commission for the Study of Ethical Problems in Medicine and Biomedical and Behavioral Research, *Defining Death: Medical, Legal, and Ethical Issues in the Determination of Death,* U.S. Government Printing Office, Washington, DC; 1981.
3. President's Commission, p. 75.
4. Julius Kerech, "Terminology, Definitions, and Usage," *Brain Death: Interrelated Medical and Social Issues,* ANYAA 9 315 1–454, The New York Academy of Sciences, 1978, p. 7.

5. President's Commission, p. 40
6. President's Commission, p. 39.
7. Senate Select Committee on the Human Embryo Experimentation Bill, 1985, *Human Embryo Experimentation in Australia,* Australia Government Public Service, 1986, p. 25.

Research with Fetal Tissue   33

The Issue

A new form of "Buck Rogers research" is well underway. Living cells taken from aborted fetuses are being transplanted into other human beings with serious diseases. Persons with Alzheimer's disease and Parkinson's disease, for example, have received transplants of brain tissue from recently aborted fetuses. The premise underlying the research is that therapy might be developed for patients with these and other debilitating diseases.

Fetal tissue is more adaptable for research, and perhaps for therapy, because fetuses do not have a well-developed immune system. Thus, the tissue garnered from fetuses is less likely to be rejected in another person's body and seems to grow faster than tissue taken from other sources. Researchers think that there is enough indication of eventual success to justify continuing the research.

Many scientists have expressed concern about ethical issues involved in this form of research because the raw material for research comes from fetuses who are killed in elective abortions. The best material for research seems to come from fetuses in the second trimester of life. As one scientist stated, "At the embryo stage, you're not just dealing with material, you're dealing with living human beings, emotions, and ethical issues; scientists are scared they won't be able to do the necessary research." Observers of the research scene are even more outspoken. A columnist in *The Wall Street Journal*, for example, called for international control of trade in fetal tissue to limit unethical procedures.

We offer the following observations as a framework for considering some of the ethical issues resulting from research with fetal tissue taken from aborted fetuses.

Ethical Reflections

1. Clearly, the research in fetal tissue has not caused the legalization of elective abortions. All know that 1.5 million abortions per year were occurring in the United States long before research with fetal tissue was initiated. For this reason, a group of lawyers, researchers, and ethicists in 1986 declared support for transplanting tissue taken from aborted fetuses.[1] At the time they stated, "We're fully aware the issue will be clouded by association with abortion, but it is important to stress we are in no way making a comment or taking a stand on the morality or legality of abortion."

The previous statement, however, does not solve all the ethical problems. Although no intrinsic connection exists between research on fetal tissue and elective abortions, those involved in this form of research have an ethical responsibility to make sure that the distance between the two realities is kept clear. There should be no indication that researchers are *promoting* elective abortion. To accomplish this, two steps should be taken:

a. No monies should be paid for fetal tissue. Some researchers and scientists have commented that they see no difficulty in using the fetal tissue from elective abortions because such abortions are legal. On the other hand, they would not approve of women becoming pregnant with the intention of having an abortion and selling the fetal tissue. Experience attests, however, that men and women in our society will do anything for money. If money can be made by becoming pregnant, then we can be assured that such a commerce will be developed. There are federal laws against the sale of organs for transplantation. It seems there should be federal laws prohibiting the sale of fetal tissue for research as well.

b. A second manner of disassociating with the destruction of living human beings is to foster the availability of fetal tissue derived from culture processes. The ethical issue resulting from the source of supply for fetal tissue might be solved if the source material for the culture is derived from spontaneous as opposed to elective abortions.

2. Although scientists are aware of the ethical issues resulting from research with fetal tissue, some consider that it is not their responsibility to grapple with these issues personally. Rather, they look to the federal government or some other agency to handle the ethical and legal issues while they continue their research. Making ethical decisions about one's work or profession is a personal responsibility. This responsibility cannot be transferred to a group of lawyers or ethicists. History demonstrates sad results when scientists renounce their personal responsibility for determining the ethical implications of their work.

3. Some ethicists and scientists compare fetal research to organ transplants from cadavers. Thus, they maintain the use of aborted fetuses is acceptable if the mother gives consent. However, further consideration belies this assumption. When a family surrenders, through proxy consent, organs from a cadaver for heart or liver transplant, they have not been involved in causing the death of the person in question. Therefore, although no direct connection exists between researchers and abortion, one cannot assume that informed consent solves the ethical issues resulting from the use of tissue from aborted fetuses.

4. Some will object to the description of elective abortion as killing a human being. One ethicist said, "Please, call it removing fetal tissue." However, it is extremely important to be clear and honest about actions under ethical analysis. This is especially true when human beings are involved. Once a group of people is deprived of their humanity, then all forms of oppression may be justified. For example, reflect on what happened to some human beings in World War II because they were designated as "non-Aryans"; think of the atrocities justified in Vietnam because Americans were fighting "Gooks"; or think about the lies and destruction of life in Central America justified because the people are identified as "Communists."

If we are to reach valid ethical solutions in healthcare and research, we must be accurate in defining the issues. The fetal tissue in this form of research comes from fetuses well along in development. Although not everyone would designate fetuses as persons to be protected fully by the law, maintaining that they are anything other than living beings and of the human species is scientifically untenable. Persons may differ as to whether any good can justify ending a human life in the early stages of development. In view of the scientific evidence, however, one has a difficult time maintaining that a fetus is anything other than a human being.

Conclusion

Research therapy with human tissue has a promising future. When assessing the ethical reasons in research and therapy, however, scientists must be concerned with more than the results. The act that produces the results must be evaluated ethically, as must the implications that follow from the action and its effects.

---

1. Mary Mahowald et al., "The Ethical Options in Transplanting Fetal Tissue," *Hastings Center Report* 7:1, February 1987, pp. 9–15.

Index

Index

GNP. *See* Gross national
product (GNP)
God, playing, 96-99
Granville, June, vii
Grave burden, 108-9, 132-33,
205
Green, Chad, 22
Gross national product (GNP),
117, 118
Guidelines, and principles, 17

Habits of the Heart, 12
Healing, and law, 100-103
Health, public, 159-70
Healthcare
corporations, investor-owned,
56-76
and decision making, 8-11,
87-90, 91-95, 145-48,
149-52, 196-97, 217-18
economics, 39-43
funding, 116-19
meaning of, 58-60
meaning and values, 61-66
Health maintenance
organization (HMO), 112-15
Helsinki Statement, 144
HIV. *See* Human immune
deficiency virus (HIV)
HMO. *See* Health maintenance
organization (HMO)
Hopelessly ill, 18
"How Patients Appraise
Physicians," 8
Human being, and death, 224
Human immune deficiency
virus (HIV), 159, 160, 161,
162, 163, 164, 165, 166, 167,
168, 169
Human life, purpose of, 120-21
Hume, David, 179
Huntington's disease, 79, 81, 82,
83
Hydration, and nutrition, 186-92

IEC. *See* Institutional ethics
committee (IEC)
Imminent death, 105-6
Inalienable rights, 56
Incompetence, 209-10
Individual liberty, and AIDS,
159-70
Informed consent, 166-67
Innate need, 69
Institutional ethics committee
(IEC), v, 21, 23, 24-25, 26,
47-48, 51-52, 53, 88-90,
145-48, 149-52, 159
Institutional review board
(IRB), 141, 143
Interaction, policy, 151
International Bioethics Summit
Conference, 31-32
Interpretation, subjective, 24-25
"Interpreting Survival Rates for
the Treatment of
Decompensated Diabetes:
Are We Saving Too Many
Lives?," 21
Investor-owned healthcare
corporations, 56-76
Investor-owned medical care
corporations, 67-73
In vitro fertilization, 32
IRB. *See* Institutional review
board (IRB)
*Issues: A Critical Examination of
Contemporary Ethical Issues
in Health Care*, v

JCAHO. *See* Joint Commission
on Accreditation of
Healthcare Organizations
(JCAHO)
Jesus, 120, 121
Jobes, Nancy Ellen, 104, 136
John Paul II, Pope, 31
Joint Commission on
Accreditation of Healthcare
Organizations (JCAHO),
193